Christ's Hospital of London, 1552–1598

Christ's Hospital of London, 1552–1598

"A Passing Deed of Pity"

Carol Kazmierczak Manzione

SUP

Selinsgrove: Susquehanna University Press
London: Associated University Presses

Associated University Presses
440 Forsgate Drive
Cranbury, NJ 08512

Associated University Presses
25 Sicilian Avenue
London WC1A 2QH, England

Associated University Presses
P.O. Box 338, Port Credit
Mississauga, Ontario
Canada L5G 4L8

The paper used in this publication meets the requirements of the American National Standard for Permanence of Paper for Printed Library Materials Z39.48-1984.

Library of Congress Cataloging-in-Publication Data

Manzione, Carol Kazmierczak, 1952–
Christ's Hospital of London, 1552–1598 : a passing deed of pity / Carol Kazmierczak Manzione.
p. cm.
Includes bibliographical references and index.
ISBN 0-945636-71-7 (alk. paper)
1. Christ's Hospital (London, England). 2. Orphanages—England--London—History. I. Title.
HV1150.L8C486 1995
362.7'32'094212—dc20 94-16865
CIP

PRINTED IN THE UNITED STATES OF AMERICA

Dedicated to my husband,
Joseph Manzione

and to the memory of my father,
Robert Kazmierczak

Contents

Preface

The purpose of this book is to examine the circumstances surrounding the foundation of Christ's Hospital and to study how this orphanage/school functioned as a charitable institution from its foundation in 1552 until the advent of the first great Elizabethan poor law in 1598. This is not intended to be a definitive study of poverty in Tudor-Stuart London or of its government; rather, it is a basic institutional study of Christ's Hospital. Neither is this intended as an exhaustive study of London in the sixteenth and seventeenth centuries; it would be redundant to recreate the excellent research done by others. In particular, Ian Archer, Paul Slack, Steven Rappaport, Paul Seaver, A. L. Beier and Roger Finalay, Jeremy Boulton, and Susan Brigden have done interesting work on this topic within the last seven years.[1]

Christ's Hospital was not established as a foundling hospital but as an orphanage and school for "the fatherless children & other poor men's children that were not able to keep them. . . ."[2] Christ's Hospital is a unique institution in that in addition to its service as an orphanage and school, it also performed as an agent of general poor relief, giving money and pensions to elderly and sick adults, even if they were childless. It appears that Christ's, in concert with St. Thomas and Bridewell, the other royal hospitals chartered by Edward VI, operated as a first line of defense against poverty in London. The government of the city of London evolved new strategies for dealing with the escalation of the problem of poverty by founding the hospitals as a systematic approach to charity administered by the government of the city of London. The foundation of the hospitals corresponded to the categories of the poor into which Tudor Englishmen were beginning to group their less fortunate countrymen: as the worthy poor and the undeserving poor. Christ's and St. Thomas hospitals were founded to treat those deemed worthy of assistance—the widows, the orphans, the sick, and the disabled. Bridewell was created to house able-bodied beggars and whores. It forced them to do honest work and tried to reform them into honest citizens.

The significance of this book is that it is not based upon childhood experiences recalled by adults or upon the diaries of a few people detailing their treatment of their own children. This study is based upon the actual treatment of a large number of children by a large number of adults.[3] One of the problems in relying upon diaries and autobiographies is that it is difficult to ascertain whether the treatment of particular children reflects larger societal attitudes or reflects the unique psychodynamic interaction between particular family members. There are too few cases to register a consistent pattern of attitude and these sources reflect mostly upper-middle-class, gentry, or aristocratic families. The children of Christ's Hospital were drawn from different classes (excluding the aristocracy, whose orphans came under the protection of the Crown). Christ's children included the offspring of the elite of the City, guildsmen, the poor, and illegitimate children. I believe that my study draws more accurate conclusions about the treatment of children in Tudor England than is possible by only relying upon literary evidence.

A standard interpretation of the treatment of children prior to the eighteenth century—the interpretation put forth by Lloyd De Mause and Lawrence Stone—maintains that they were commonly mistreated by their parents.[4] As will be shown, Christ's Hospital gave loving, compassionate care to its charges. If such comparative strangers treated the children well, are we to conclude that their own parents and relations routinely abused and neglected them?

This study draws heavily upon the official records of Christ's Hospital: the formal records of the minutes from the meetings of the governors, the audited account books, and the children's register. It suffers from the limitations of those sources. It is known what decisions were reached in the minutes of meetings, for instance, but not necessarily the process involved in reaching those decisions. The City records and company records were also consulted, but generally provided little additional information.

This book is divided into a introduction and six chapters. The introduction examines the conditions of poverty affecting the capital. The first chapter traces the foundation and circumstances surrounding Christ's beginning. Chapter 2 describes the administration and complex structure of the hospital. Chapters 3 and 4 analyze its fiscal situation; the former details the sources of revenue and the latter Christ's expenditures. Chapter 5 discusses the governors and chapter 6 the children.

I have modernized spelling and punctuation. First names have been changed to modern spellings, but I have left last names unchanged. Dates remain in Old Style. I have also converted roman numerals into arabic numbers.

I am indebted to the following for encouragement: Edwin and Anne Dewindt, Daniel Bjork, Carole Levine, Jackie Murray, Paul Seaver, Vanessa Harding, Valerie Pearl, Majorie McIntere, Jackie Zeff, Carol Weisfeld, and Sister Gilmary Bauer. David Young, the archivist of Christ's Hospital, has been a wonderful support throughout the long years of research. The staff of the Guildhall Library and the Corporation of London Record Office provided friendly and indispensable assistance and they have my most humble thanks. Lastly, I am grateful to the faculty of Mercy College of Detroit for the summer research grant they awarded me in the summer of 1991 to fine-tune my research.

Christ's Hospital
of London,
1552–1598

Introduction: London in 1552

London, thou art of towns *A per se.*
Sovereign of cities, seemliest in sight,
Of high renown, riches, and royalty;
Of lords, barons, and many goodly knight;
Of most delectable lusty ladies bright;
Of famous prelates in habits clerical;
Of merchants full of substance and might:
London, thou art the flower of Cities all.

—William Dunbar (1501)

Dignity – "Was there ever in any age the like number of poor people as there are at this present begging in the streets of the City and wandering in the fields so idly, being ready to attempt any mischief upon any light occasion"?
Duty – "The number at this present is great & yet in times past much greater."

—John Howes (1582)

The poem by William Dunbar, quoted above, was written to honor London and reflects the new sense of pride and prosperity that its citizens were beginning to experience under the first of the Tudors, Henry VII. London was assuming a prominence and leadership in English affairs that would grow and strengthen. John Howes, reflecting upon London in 1582, saw a different city, one that was beginning to show the strain of unprecedented growth. These two opinions of London in less than a hundred years describe a crucial time for the City. One historian characterized these years as

> a turning-point for London. Until then, it had been a town on the outer edge of the large net of European trade, now it became the centre of the still larger one which was to spread over continents.[1]

The sixteenth century that began to bring to London the blessings of growth also brought the problems of poverty, disease, and overcrowding. For not the last time, London would become infamous for her slums. As the century wore on and London's expansion continued unchecked, there was an increased focus on the problem caused by that growth, namely, poverty.

The first half of the sixteenth century saw the increasing pauperization of the majority of the population, who had always lived on the edge of bare subsistence. The years from 1510 to 1552 were years of crisis for England, and whatever happened in England was reflected and intensified in London.[2] There were several changes in the economic structure of England that caused an increase in paupers and especially paupers on the move. It was these vagrants who posed such a problem for town officials, who saw them as a criminal threat. In Tudor England, men and woman were no longer tied securely in one place by the medieval manorial system, but were free to move to seek their fortunes. London beckoned like a shining light, which held a promise of hope and a last resort to the desperate. Like all cities, it was a place of contrast and diversity. There were extremes of poverty and wealth, debauchery and holiness. For some, London provided the advantages of a great metropolis: freedom, economic success, and anonymity. "To the ambitious it has offered preferment, to the distressed a promise, more often unfulfilled than not, of employment and perhaps of wealth."[3] Indeed, more often than not, London proved to be less than a paradise:

> Whereas medieval migration usually involved respectable people becoming apprentices in the city gilds, many immigrants between 1500 and 1700 were the poor and destitute, who journeyed to London in desperate hope of casual work or charity, and who crowded the small tenements of poor parishes or squatted in suburban slums.[4]

John Pound, in *Poverty and Vagrancy in Tudor England*, sees a complex interaction between eight factors that amplified the problem of poverty, of which begging was the most visible manifestation.[5] These eight factors were roving retainers and ex-servicemen, the rising population,[6] the fluctuations in the cloth industry, enclosures of farmland,[7] inflation,[8] plague,[9] agricultural fluctuations,[10] and the dissolution of the monasteries.[11] None of these conditions alone could have caused poverty of the extent that the sixteenth century witnessed. However, the combination of these factors was deadly.

Of course, poverty was not a new problem, but some of the factors contributing to poverty were new. The most important new force, and the most crucial for London, was an increase in population after over a century-and-a-half of negligible growth. The last big population surge had occurred around 1300. After the decimation of the English population by the Black Death, it took England until around 1520 to begin to recover its pre-plague population. It is impossible to give precise population figures before the advent of the National Census in 1801, but crude estimates are possible. The population of England doubled between 1500 and 1700, and this growth was greater than that of any other European country. England grew by over 110 percent, while Europe as a whole increased by an estimated 42 percent.[12] Julian Cornwall, in his article "English Population in the Early Sixteenth Century," estimates that the population of England was 2.3 million in 1522–25; 2.8 million in 1545; and 3.75 million in 1603.[13] John Hatcher, in *Plague, Population and the English Economy, 1348-1530,* believes that Cornwall's figure of 2.3 million may be too low and proposes 2.25 to 2.75 million in 1522–25 as a more accurate figure.[14] More recently, Wrigley and Schofield place the population at 2,773,851 in 1541, 2,853,711 in 1546, and 3,011,030 in 1551.[15] Although there is debate among scholars about the exact numbers, no one disagrees that the population of England was growing in the sixteenth century.

As impressive as England's growth was, the growth of London was even more spectacular. Half of the urban growth from 1500 to 1700 was due to the growth of London.[16] By 1700, metropolitan London contained about 10 percent of England's population.[17] The growth of London cannot be explained by an overall growth in urbanization, because London held in 1520 more than five times the number of inhabitants as the next largest city, Norwich. By 1603, metropolitan London held more than thirteen times as many people as Norwich.[18] The city grew both absolutely and in comparison with other English towns. In 1500, London possessed around fifty thousand people; by 1550 it had a population of seventy thousand, and would possess around two hundred thousand by the end of the century.[19] In less than a hundred years, London had more than quadrupled her population, an incredible rate of growth. The growth of the capital was due not to a high birth rate among its citizens, but due to immigration from other regions of England. Most of these new residents were poor. "A substantial part of the metropolitan population was poor, often recruited from the countryside."[20]

Tudor London held the largest single concentration of population in England and was rapidly outgrowing the older mechanisms for dealing with the needy at a time of great economic dislocation. Henry VIII's statute of 1531, a legislative attempt to eliminate beggary, expresses very well the threat that officials felt.

> Where in all places throughout this realm of England, vagabonds and beggars have of long time increased and daily do increase in great and excessive numbers by the occasion of idleness, mother and root of all vices, whereby hath insurged and sprung and daily insurgeth and springeth continual thefts, murders, and other heinous offenses and great enormities to the high displeasure of God, the inquietation and damage of the king's people, and to the marvelous disturbance of the common weal of this realm.[21]

The problem seems to have alarmed officials, who predicted horrible consequences if it was not immediately brought under control by passing laws, rules, and regulations—a quick and tidy way to deal with any problem. In 1552, John Howes, echoing the attitude of other Londoners, attributed the current crisis to "want of execution of good laws & by negligent government. . . ."[22] Clearly, a complex situation such as poverty could not be solved even if enlightened laws were enacted and enforced by dedicated officials. However ineffective, controlling beggars by simply making begging illegal was a tactic that was tried again and again, each time making the penalties more gruesome.

> Because vagrants appeared to present a threat to the state, Tudor governments indulged in an orgy of attempts to crush them that included refusal of alms, whipping, stocking, imprisonment, branding, ear boring, forced labour in the galleys, slavery, deportation and hanging. Constructive efforts to solve the problem by setting vagrants to work were small waves in this sea of corporal punishment.[23]

In 1552, the year of the foundation of the royal hospitals (of which Christ's was one), there was widespread concern that the public order was being undermined by beggars. The Common Council also concluded in 1552 that the "great number of beggars, vagabonds, idle and suspect persons [had] increased within this city and the commonwealth thereby [was] much impaired, and evil rule much enhanced and grown, and the ability and surety of the said city much decreased and diminished."[24] A suit sent to the Privy Council by the citizens of London in the same year forcibly states "that it was too evident to all men that beggary and thievery did abound. . . ."[25] The urban government seemed to believe they were literally being besieged by the poor and that their numbers were larger than ever, increasing, and would soon be out of control without active, immediate intervention. The city officials seemed desperate to clean up the streets and tried to think of ways that

> these great numbers of idle roguish wandering beggers might be removed out of the streets & every sort placed in sundry houses the young the aged the sore & the lusty rogue & every of these to be made profitable members in the common wealth.[26]

Who exactly were these vagrants that so terrorized the psyche of Tudor Englishman? A. L. Beier's article "Vagrants and the Social Order in Elizabethan England" documents the composition of vagrants based upon arrest records and contradicts some ideas that Londoners held about the nature of the beast threatening their municipal order. There is no evidence that vagrants were organized into criminal bands to terrorize honest citizens.[27] According to Beier, the majority of vagrants were single men and single women who had previously been employed in such unstable occupations as laborers, servants, and cloth workers.[28]

Was Tudor London swamped with the poor and needy? D. M. Palliser has observed that the problem of poverty "was a major preoccupation of contemporaries, a preoccupation reflected in voluminous statutes, by-laws and accounts. Yet it would be misleading to conclude that it was as serious and growing a problem. . . ."[29] In 1552, a blue-ribbon committee appointed to look into the problem found that there were 2110 respectable needy.[30] Even if this figure was too low and it is doubled to cover the undeserving poor, it still represents only around 6 percent. This number indicates there was no invasion of destitute needy. But while the total number of poor people might not be impressive, the people themselves were visible and inescapable on the streets of London, and to local officials they were omnipresent. They also came to symbolize transition and change. They were perceived to represent a new problem, and one that might not be readily resolvable. These people represented to the establishment the potential breakdown of the social order at a time when the strain of religious discord and economic instability threatened to rend English society in the way it was rending societies on the Continent. Moreover, the poor were no longer just the deserving poor, but those who were on the fringes of society. Paul Slack makes the following astute observation about the marginality of these new poor:

> The simplest way of defending virtue and order was by defining vice and disorder. . . .The use of the poor as a yardstick, against which approved social norms could be measured out, may be seen most clearly in the representation of vagrants and idle paupers as the complete obverse of all that was acceptable.[31]

Examining the attitudes toward charity, and how the undeserving poor came to be separated and distinguished from the deserving poor, provides insight into the fears and hopes of a society beginning its transformation into a modern urban center.

Attitudes toward Charity

> to set the poor on work, that there should be houses of correction built in all counties, and stock in money provided, to set all the poor (that can work) or lack work, to spin, knit, or such like, (and all the impotent to be otherwise relieved by weekly contribution).
>
> —Henry Arthington (1597)

Charitable works performed by religious houses in England had included tending to the sick, giving food and money to the poor, and taking care of the outcasts of society, such as lepers and abandoned babies. The dissolution of the monasteries and convents that occurred between 1536 and 1540 destroyed the religious houses but provided no alternative for tending to the needy; it had removed the only place where the needy had been helped. The Reformation began a shift away from the abuses of Catholic Church, especially those institutions eschewing the virtues of poverty—the monasteries and convents. Their removal served to amplify a crisis of poverty. While the effectiveness of the charity mechanism of the Catholic Church could be questioned, it is beyond dispute that the church had been the primary agency performing acts of charity and its institutions had been put out of existence at a time when the need was great.

> It fell to secular authority to provide help for the poor. Their dissolution meant that reform of poor relief in sixteenth-century England was not a matter simply of re-organizing or supplementing existing provision. . . . It required intervention by secular authorities and individual donors to replace what had been lost and thus, it must often have seemed, to rebuild a system of social welfare from scratch.[32]

The influx of destitute people who had little chance of obtaining permanent employment added a new dimension to the problem of urban poverty; they weren't provincials who were going to be apprenticed to a member of one of the city companies. Many of these people didn't belong to the urban corporations that were characteristic of earlier urban life. It was one thing to help the widow and children of a fellow guild member, someone known to you, and quite another to help strangers, who had no ties to the community and therefore no real place in that society. Charity moved from being limited aid through a life crisis to being a long-term arrangement. This left many poor people without a place to turn for help, and the guilds and the churches could no longer provide the bulk of the aid.

Who exactly were the poor and needy? The sixteenth century began to sort the poor into the general categories of the deserving and undeserving.

> Distinction was made between the aged, impotent poor and the beggars and vagabonds. Of the latter those willing to work were to be given work, the unwilling were to be punished for their medieval sin of idleness. The problem confronting Tudor statesmen was to devise machinery for assisting those deserving aid or willing to work and for punishing the indolent.[33]

The distinction between those who were needy because of circumstances beyond their control, such as illness or old age, and those who were poor because of their own laziness or moral defect came to have increasing importance: the former were to be relieved and the later were to be punished and set to work.[34]

> The deserving and undeserving could be distinguished by their behaviour and moral worth, and while the first were relieved by alms, or later by public rates, the second could be whipped without compunction, sent back to their home parishes and compelled to work there.[35]

There was a further breakdown of the poor into three categories:

> [A]ll the poor were divided into three parts: the poor by impotency, being the orphans, the aged, the crippled and the blind; the poor by casualty, the sick, diseased, and wounded; the thriftless poor, rogues, vagabonds and whores.[36]

The citizens of London in a petition to the king divided the poor thusly:

And among the whole rout of needy and miserable persons, we espied three sundry sorts which were diversely to be provided for; the succourless poor child, the sick and impotent, the sturdy vagabond, or idle person.[37]

Clearly the English were beginning to make important moral distinctions about the poor. Pre-Reformation society had a long history of tending to needy children and to other unfortunate people, and there was a patient acceptance of poverty as being Christlike. Giving alms to the poor was an opportunity of atoning for sins and saving one's soul. Reformation society began to perceive poor people as a threat to the social order and began to see poverty, not as a estate to bring one closer to God by denying earthly needs, but as a punishment from God for sinfulness.

The abolition of the religious orders at the Reformation removed the need to admit the holiness of voluntary poverty altogether; and Protestant invective against monks and friars insisted that poverty must never be actively sought.[38]

Henry Arthington, whose elaborate description and evaluation of the poor has already been partially quoted, also strongly condemns those who fall into the group of sturdy beggars for bringing this condition upon themselves. He says they should not be pitied.

[T]he reason is, for that they do not complain unto God of their grievous sins. . . . First, that they have misspent much good time in idle roguing up and own, and would not work. . . . Second, that in time of abundance, they have been great wasters. . . .Thirdly, that when God by his messengers, called upon them to leave their evil ways, and serve him better, they would not hear. . . .[39]

In short, if the poor refused to work, then they must be forced to labor for the good of their souls and the commonwealth.

It therefore became easier to deny help altogether to the unworthy poor, for they were dangerous and assisting them undermined the security of society. The modern social welfare system bureaucratized with complex rules and regulations for determining eligibility had its roots in Tudor perceptions. "Discrimination and public relief made it necessary to define private charity, and in the process it became exclusive, calculating and deliberate. . . ."[40]

The foundation of the royal hospitals constituted a new charitable approach to the problem of poverty and an attempt to go beyond repressive legislation that was difficult, if not impossible, to enforce. The royal hospitals were jointly founded by royal proclamation, funded by private citizens, and administrated by municipal authority. It was a unique arrangement that was divorced from clerical control and administered through the civil government of the city of London. The intention of the leadership of London was to reform some of the conditions causing poverty, and that was a new attitude. Poverty was not a God-given condition that was sometimes alleviated by the generosity of Christians, but was a human condition that could be challenged by man.

> Central to relief in the capital were the hospitals founded in the mid-Tudor period on a wave of godly enthusiasm and alarm about the growing dimensions of London's poverty. They represented a comprehensive approach to the problem, categorizing the poor in terms of the sick and impotent who were to be cared for in St Thomas' and St Bartholomew's, orphaned children who became the responsibility of Christ's, the unemployed and work-shy who were to be set to work or disciplined in Bridewell, and decayed householders relieved by pensions raised through the poor rate.[41]

The royal hospitals did not function in the same manner as their medieval predecessors; they operated not as alms-giving institutions spewing charity right and left but as a mechanism for social change through education and hard work. "[T]he humanists were extolling education as a panacea for the ills of the body politic . . . moral reformers of the period expressed the hope that schooling could be used to combat such social vices as idleness and unruliness."[42]

Londoners were redefining not only their relationship to God but society as a whole, and meant to create a Christian commonwealth.

> The reformers had looked to the advent of a Christian commonwealth with the dissolution of the religious houses; not only would monastic abuses be removed, they hoped, but monastic wealth would be distributed to the poor.[43]

Paul Slack wisely cautions against drawing too fine a line between Catholic and Protestant approaches to charity. "We must conclude that we can point to few clear-cut or lasting distinctions between Catholic and

Protestant approaches to social welfare."[44] It wasn't the new Protestant theology that was as crucial as the freeing of wealth that had previously belonged to the Catholic Church. With the dissolution of the religious houses, it allowed for the re-allocation of property and resources and placed some of them into the hands of the merchants and craftsmen of London, who were very careful with their newfound responsibilities. However, it would be an error to conclude that the dynamism of the new Church of England had nothing to do with the foundation of the royal hospitals; these men expressed their motivations and efforts in the vocabulary of religion. Part of the charge given to the governors after their annual election meeting underscores a profound belief that they were doing God's work and that dire consequences would follow inadequate service.

> {Y]our charge shall be in this government, that every of you endeavor yourselves with all your wisdom and powers faithfully and diligently to serve in this vocation and calling; which is an office of high trust and worship; for ye are called to be the faithful and true distributors and disposer of the goods of Almighty God to his poor and needy members.[45]

The City rulers saw their efforts at poor relief as carrying out a directive from God and emphasized their stewardship. Philip Gavitt observes there was a similar attitude in Renaissance Florence: "the notion of earthly goods as goods entrusted to the testator by his Creator, and thus to be conceived of and used for the improvement and salvation of the testator's soul."[46]

The motivation for the foundation of Christ's Hospital, as well as of St. Thomas, St. Bartholomew's, and Bridewell, is to be found in the belief that there was a crisis of poverty, that the City could manage the crisis, that education could reform social conditions, and that God blessed their efforts. The creation of the hospitals reflects a fortunate convergence of Protestant piety and efficient municipal administration. How this partnership came into existence and the dramatic story of the foundation of the royal hospitals provides the focus of the next chapter.

1
The Solution: The Royal Hospitals

I.

> They [the merchant elite] represent the first really significant advance towards the assumption of civic responsibility for the cure of illness and the care of completely helpless persons.
>
> —W. K. Jordan, *The Charities of London: 1480–1660*

> Requiring everyone of you faithfully to travail in this your office and calling; that this work may have his perfection, and that the needy number committed to your charge be diligently and wholesomely provided for. And for your care towards these poor and needy members of Christ, you shall be rewarded at his hand, and receive his blessing in this world, and in the world to come the joys everlasting.
>
> —Charge given to the governors of the royal hospitals

Although Christ's Hospital, St. Thomas, and Bridewell were founded together, they functioned as independent establishments and each merits study in its own right. They served different needs because they were founded to counter different problems. Each hospital had its own set of governors who ran their own hospital without interference from the governors of the other hospitals. Additionally, each had its own source of income and dispensed its own revenue. Notwithstanding the autonomy, there was some overlapping between personnel, gifts, and money. Every year on or around the feast of St. Matthew (21 September), the governors and officials of all royal hospitals would hold a general meeting at Christ's Hospital to select new officials and governors, or reappoint those already serving.[1] Although this study is concerned primarily with the foundation and operation of Christ's Hospital, a brief discussion of St. Thomas and Bridewell is important to an understanding of the role of Christ's in the urban environment of Tudor London.

St. Thomas the Apostle Hospital, located across the Thames in Southwark, was founded as a place to tend to the needy and sick of London—in other words to act as a hospital in the modern sense of the word. St. Thomas received the following charge:

> There was also devised to be taken out of the streets all the lame and aged people such as had not any place to go unto. And they should all be conveyed to the Hospital of St. Thomas in Southwark where they should have meat, drink, and lodging, Surgeons and other officers to attend upon them.[2]

This responsibility to tend to the sick had been partially fulfilled prior to the Dissolution. St. Thomas had been founded around 1106, and was known as The Hospital of St. Thomas the Martyr, having been named after St. Thomas Becket after his death in 1173.[3] It was dissolved in 1540 and was evaluated as being worth £266 17s 6d. It reopened as a hospital in 1552, and acquired the new name of St. Thomas the Apostle Hospital, because Becket had been decanonized.[4] "St. Thomas in Southwark being an Hospital of great receipt for the poor, was suppressed, but again newly founded and endowed by the benevolence and charity of the citizens of London."[5] Unlike Christ's and Bridewell, then, St. Thomas was not a new creation. It was not so much founded as refounded in 1552.

The founding of the third royal hospital, Bridewell, came about in a different manner from the other two. It came into existence as the result of a distinct request by the citizens of London to the king in 1552, when they asked that "the King's highness's house of Bridewell" be used as a "house of occupations."[6] John Stow, whose *Survey of London* is the most used and respected source for information on sixteenth-century London, described it as "Bridewell, now an Hospital (or house of correction) founded by King Edward the Sixth, to be a Workhouse for the poor and idle persons of the City, wherein a great number of vagrant persons be now set awork, and relieved at the charges of the citizens."[7] Bridewell was originally built in 1515–20 as a palace for Henry VIII on the banks of the Fleet River close to Blackfriars Monastery. Bridewell seems to have stopped serving as a royal residence beginning in 1531, when it was leased to the French ambassador.[8] However royal its former occupants, Bridewell Hospital was created to be a workhouse and to force the beggars off the streets. According to John Howes:

> Then they did devise that all the idle & lusty rogues as well as women should all be taken up & be conveyed into some house where they should have all things necessary & be compelled to labour.[9]

The establishment of Bridewell represented a new departure in official policy toward the poor. The recipients of the charity of this hospital were not sick, disabled, old, or children, the worthy objects of traditional Christian charity, but able-bodied men and women quite capable of working. These people were believed by the authorities to be inclined to idleness out of perversity and, as we have already seen, secular authority viewed these beggars not as unfortunate people but as a threat to society.

The three royal hospitals became four with the refounding of St. Bartholomew's at some time between 26 June 1553 and the first recorded minutes of the Court of Governors of Christ's on 27 September 1557.[10] It soon became interwoven through finances and governors with the others.

St. Bart's, like St. Thomas, was a place of medical care. It had been originally founded in 1123 by an Augustinian named Rahere and was dissolved in 1537 by Henry VIII.[11] "The priory and hospital at the time of the Dissolution possessed net revenues of £304 16s 5d p. a."[12] St. Bart's is located in Smithfield, just north, beyond the city wall, from Christ's Hospital. "St. Bartolomew in Smithfield, an Hospital of great receipt and relief for the poor, was suppressed by Henry the Eight, and again by him given to the City, and is endowed by the Citizen's benevolence."[13] St. Bart's was refounded by Henry VIII in 1544 and the citizens of London agreed to raise 500 pounds annually to support it and Bethlem Hospital, which had also been given back to the City.[14]

> The Hospital of St Bartholomew's is the only one of the mediaeval hospitals of London still to occupy the original site of its foundation. . . . Then, on 27 December [1544], Henry signed with his own hand the first document of refoundation, an indenture between himself and the City in which he gave to the mayor and commonalty and citizens of London and their successors for ever "the late hospital of St Bartholomew." . . . On 13 January 1547, a fortnight before he died, Henry completed the work by issuing, under the great seal of England . . .[15]

St. Bart's is frequently omitted from discussion when talking about the hospitals, possibly due to its later addition and because it was not part of the original charter and that it was already functioning as a hospital before the creation of the other hospitals in 1552. It is to the foundation of Christ's Hospital that we now turn.

II.

> Christ's Hospital erected was a passing deed of pity.
>
> —Poem under a stained glass window in the former Governor's Meeting Room

> But the foundation of Christ's Hospital was such an unique example of the co-operation between men of faith and good will in an act of Christian charity.
>
> —Edmund Blunden, *The Christ's Hospital Book*

The function of Christ's Hospital was more complicated than that of the other hospitals. Christ's not only served as an orphanage but also as a school and as an agent for poor relief. It may seem strange that this orphanage pensioned the elderly and disabled; however, this makes a great deal of sense if one remembers the classifications of the poor at that time: the sick, who were cared for at St. Thomas and St. Bartholomew's; the lusty beggars, who were forced to work and hopefully reformed at Bridewell; and the rest of the honest poor, the disabled, orphans, and elderly, who were served by Christ's. Therefore, this orphanage functioned as a place to assist the respectable poor who were not ill, whether or not they were parents. We will examine this unusual clientele in more detail in later chapters.

Christ's Hospital's role as an orphanage was not an innovation, for the citizens of London had a long tradition of caring for its orphans: this "passing deed of pity" did not suddenly materialize but drew upon the customs and practices of the City of London. The foundation of Christ's Hospital as an orphanage involved its assumption of some elements of three traditional practices established by the City: the Court of Orphans; the regulation of apprentices; and the charge of the hospitals formerly under the pale of the dissolved religious orders.[16]

The first municipal practice involved the City's assumption of the legal right to appoint guardians for the orphaned children of freemen of the City of London. This practice had in fact been long institutionalized through the Court of Orphans. Charles Carlton's book on the court traces its institutional origins from its establishment in 1276 through its formalization as the Court of Orphans two centuries later.[17] However, this institution was fully developed by the time of the Tudors and followed a set procedure in assuming responsibility for individual children:

> The mayor was informed of the death of any freeman by the constables of the city. These officials were required to certify each month

> to the clerk of the mayor's court the names of any freeman who had died within his precinct, as well as the names of his children. The common crier then summoned the widow or executor to appear before the court of the Lord Mayor and aldermen to bring an inventory of the testator's estate.[18]

It must be emphasized that the term *orphan* does not refer to parentless children, but to fatherless children. In Tudor London, a child could be an orphan and have a mother still alive. Thus, in a suit by the citizens of London requesting that the former palace of Bridewell be given to the City for a hospital, they refer to "Christ's Hospital, which is the house of the fatherless. . . ."[19] John Howes, who wrote an account of the foundation of Christ's Hospital in 1582, thereby providing an irreplaceable source of information on the early history of the hospital, described it as a place for "the fatherless children."[20] Conversely, a motherless child was not considered an orphan. The Lord Mayor's duty in cases of a fatherless child was to make a complete summary of the property of the deceased citizen to ensure that the minor heir would not be cheated and to appoint a guardian for the child. The responsibility did not, however, end there:

> Once they had granted an orphan's wardship, the mayor and aldermen had two main responsibilities: first, to ensure that during his minority the child was properly fed, housed, clothed and educated; and, second, to see that the guardian safely kept the orphan's inheritance, and paid it to the child when he came of age.[21]

And indeed, these goals would be similar to those set forth in the Letters Patent (26 June, 7 Edward VI, 1553) that incorporated Christ's Hospital, wherein King Edward VI states "that by such reason and care neither children yet being in their infancy shall lack good education and instruction nor when they shall obtain riper years shall be destitute of honest callings and occupations. . . ."[22]

The City had therefore assumed the legal responsibility for tending to the orphans of the freemen of London, and that was institutionalized in the Court of Orphans. However, by the sixteenth century the problem was not limited to City orphans but encompassed abandoned and deserted children as well. These deserted children were not only the offspring of London citizens; often they were born elsewhere and came to London with their parents. Some of these parents came to seek employment in the City, and failing to support themselves or their children felt compelled to abandon them. Sometimes, illegitimate infants were deliberately brought to London to be abandoned. Not only were the numbers of orphans increasing, but more of them fell under categories beyond those for which the Court of Orphans had traditionally assumed responsibility, namely freeman of the City and their dependents. The founding of Christ's Hospital was in part a response to this admixture of quantitative increase and qualitative divergence.

The second municipal practice, overseeing the regulations of apprentices, would become an important aspect of the operation of Christ's Hospital. To avoid the possibility that children under its care would become permanently dependent on charity, the functions of Christ's Hospital were closely tied to the existing apparatus of municipally regulated apprenticeships. When the boys and girls reached the ages of fourteen to fifteen and were thus eligible for formal apprenticeship, they had not only been cared for in a general sense but had also been prepared educationally and morally for that position.

The third municipal practice was London's assumption, after the dissolution of the monasteries in 1536–38, of the control over the hospitals dedicated to care for the sick and needy.[23] The suppression of monasteries and convents was part of the wholesale confiscation of church property during the English Reformation.[24] Former church properties were sold or given to Henry VIII's powerful subjects. The transition of church lands to private property played a part in the rapid growth of London during the sixteenth century.[25] The gardens and grounds attached to religious houses provided the land needed for housing of the growing population and produced a significant profit to the new owners. London's growth also brought with it the problems of poverty and abandoned children, stretching the available resources. Therefore Christ's Hospital was created as a municipal institution to insure that the children were not only fed, clothed, and housed, but also educated to be good, useful, and productive citizens of the City. The governors themselves spoke of this goal in their minutes of 27 September 1557 when they declared, "Christ's Hospital hath been erected for the virtuous bringing up of the miserable youth. . . ."[26]

Although the successful push for the establishment of Christ's Hospital was made in the reign of Edward VI, these efforts had really started during the reign of Henry VIII, Edward's father, who had donated Greyfriars to the City. Greyfriars, a Franciscan monastery, had been abandoned after its suppression on 12 November 1538, and was not utilized effectively either for private or public purpose until it became the home of Christ's

Hospital. After it was suppressed, Greyfriars served briefly, in 1544, as a storehouse for loot from the war with France.[27] Ironically, the former monastery was itself looted of its valuables, a not uncommon practice with former church properties. After its brief use as a storehouse, Greyfriars "stood void & empty" before its transformation into Christ's Hospital.[28] Greyfriars was located in the ward of Farringdon Within in the northwest part of the City, just inside Newgate. The monastery bordered on the city wall to the north and the west and on Newgate Market to the south. Greyfriars housed the tombs of numerous distinguished persons, including three queens. Buried there were Queen Margaret, wife of Edward I; Queen Isabell, wife of Edward II; and Queen Joanna, wife to David II of Scotland.[29] Sometime after 1545, anything and everything of value was taken out and sold, including the tomb marble:

> for there were 9 tombs of alabaster and marble, inured with strikes of iron in the choir, and one tomb in the body of the Church, also coped with iron, all pulled down, besides seven-score grave stones of marble, all sold for 50 pounds, or thereabouts, by Sir Martin Bowes, Goldsmith and Alderman of London.[30]

This same Sir Martin Bowes, Lord Mayor of London and undertreasurer of the royal mint in 1545, when he acted as the agent for the sale of the marble, became the president of Christ's Hospital for a short time in 1556.[31] He would also become the comptroller general for the four hospitals from 1556 until 1566.

In addition to being known for its tombs, Greyfriars Monastery was also famous for its library. It is somehow fitting that in its second life as Christ's Hospital, the tradition of scholarship would continue. The library was over a hundred years old and housed a sizable collection of books:

> Richard Whittington in the year 1429 founded the library, which was in length one hundred twenty-nine feet, and in breadth thirty-one: all sealed with wainscot, having twenty-eight desks, and eight double settles of wainscot. Which in the next year following was altogether finished in building, and within three years after, furnished with books, to the charges of five hundred fifty-six pound, ten shillings, whereof Richard Whittington bare four hundred pound. . . .[32]

Greyfriars was given to the Lord Mayor and citizens of London on 27 December 1547 by Henry VIII. Specifically, he gave to the Lord Mayor and citizens of London "the Greyfriars Church, with all the edifices & ground, the Fratrie, the Library, the Dortar, & Chapterhouse, [and] the great Cloistery. . . ."[33] This same agreement gave St. Bartholomew's Hospital to the City. This deed of covenant additionally reorganized the parish structure in that part of London. The church of Greyfriars became a regular parish church, which would count the inhabitants of Christ's Hospital as part of its flock and would be the place where the children would regularly worship:

> The Grey friars' church renamed Christchurch, became parochial, its parish including those of St. Nicholas, St. Ewen, and the part of St. Sepulchre's within the Wall, and also the children and officers of Christ's Hospital, and the other inhabitants of that precinct; it was served by a vicar appointed and paid a fixed salary by the City.[34]

After obtaining control of Greyfriars, the City lost interest in its further use. London officials may have thought that because St. Bart's was again functioning as a hospital shortly after its being handed over to the City in 1547, there was no urgency related to the provision of another hospital. However, with only one hundred beds, St. Bart's was clearly overwhelmed by the number of poor people needing care.[35] Money was not forthcoming for additional hospitals. The City already had the buildings of Greyfriars—it needed to provide the "matching funds." Eventually, five years later, that monetary support would materialize and make possible the preparation of Greyfriars to accept children under the new name of Christ's Hospital in 1552. The reason why the need for more hospitals for the poor was not felt before 1552 may be related to the attempt by the Crown to control the problem by passage of new poor laws in 1547 and 1549; the 1547 law allowed for slavery of people who refused to work.[36] By 1552, it was obvious that legislative action was not effective and the problem had not been alleviated but had escalated.

The transformation of the empty Greyfriars into Christ's Hospital is a rather dramatic story. First, it was chartered only days before the death of the sixteen-year-old king, Edward Tudor, himself an orphan. The Letters Patent were signed on 26 June 1553 and he died on July 6 of the same year. King Edward was aware of the numbers of poor people who were causing such concern to the citizens of the City of London and he spoke in the Charter of "pitying the miserable estate of the poor, fatherless, decrepit, aged, sick and infirm and impotent persons, languishing under various kind of diseases. . . ."[37] According to Howes and the uncritically accepted explanation, this general awareness on the part of the king was converted into action through the influence of a sermon given at Whitehall in January 1552 by Nicholas Ridley, bishop of London.[38]

> [I]n a sermon before the king's majesty [he] did so zealously move the king to have a care for the relief of the poor that the king after the end of the sermon sent for the Bishop & conferred with him what course might best be taken for the relief of the poor.[39]

Howes to the contrary, Edward was not struck by a bolt of homiletic lightning and moved to establish hospitals without ever having given prior thought to the problem of poverty besetting his kingdom. As we have seen, the poverty crisis had been in existence since the 1520s and had amplified greatly by the time of Edward's reign. Edwardian poor laws, like the Henrician poor laws of 1531 and 1536, oscillated between severity and attempts to look at the root causes of the poverty problem.[40]

After the conference between Edward and Ridley, the king gave him letters to turn over to the Lord Mayor, Sir Richard Dodd, commanding action. (It was this Sir Richard Dodd "[w]hose picture . . . his friends [had] set, to put each wight in mind, to imitate his virtuous deeds. . . .")[41] Sir Richard Dodd, the Lord Mayor of London in 1552, was instrumental in the creation of Christ's Hospital. Thirty men, both aldermen and citizens, formed a committee to oversee the project. "So that after divers meeting of the Bishop and otherwise Citizens they devised a book wherein they had set down in what sort and manner they would have these poor provided for."[42] The committee requested that the aldermen make a search cf their wards and submit the number of "fatherless children . . . sore & sick persons . . . poor men overburdened with their children . . . aged persons . . . decayed householders . . . and idle vagabonds."[43]

After the committee had identified and classified the needy into groups, the gathering of funds began in earnest. They started with themselves and donated approximately 548 pounds.[44] The committee's fund-raising efforts bear some similarities to modern methods of raising money for charity. The committee began to publicize the need for money by using the mass medium of the day, the pulpit. "And to that effect they delivered there with a very fine witty and learned oration being printed which they gave to every preacher and minister the better to instruct and persuade the people in every parish to give liberally."[45] They even distributed what we would call pledge cards for "every man to set down his own name and his sum what he would give presently and weekly."[46] Boxes were also placed around the City, especially in churches and public buildings, for the purpose of collecting the random coins of pious worshippers. The citizens of London responded with charitable enthusiasm. Between Christmas 1552 and midsummer 1554, the hospitals of Christ's and St. Thomas received over six thousand pounds.[47]

The repairs to the buildings that had been Greyfriars began in late spring 1552. Clearly, little maintenance could have been done on Greyfriars after its suppression as a monastery, and these buildings must have been in a deplorable condition. Over £326 was spent in 1552 and 1553 to make the buildings inhabitable for the children. The work to prepare Greyfriars to become Christ's Hospital moved rather quickly and in less than a year after Ridley's speech the first children were admitted.

> [T]o make short, every man granted liberally, according to his ability, books were drawn of the relief in every ward of the City, towards the new hospitals, and were delivered by the Mayor to the King's Commissioners, on the 17 of February, and order was taken therein, so as the 26 of July, in the year 1552. The repairing of the Greyfriars house, for poor fatherless children, was taken in hand. . . .[48]

By November of 1552, the transformation of the old monastery into Christ's Hospital had been completed.

> [T]he citizens proceeded vigorously with the necessary repairs of the old conventual edifice, which in less than six months had sufficiently advanced to allow of the admission of three hundred and forty children in the month of November. . . .[49]

The children would make their first public appearance, a month after their installation, at Christmas. This appearance on a major holiday established a tradition. Each year the children would attend the annual Easter sermon given at St. Mary Spital, which is located near Bishopsgate; it was delivered in a churchyard pulpit called the Spital (or Spittle) Cross.[50]

> On Christmas day in the afternoon, while the Lord Mayor and aldermen rode to Paul's [St. Paul's Cathedral], the children of Christ's Hospital stood, from Saint Lawrence Lane end in Cheap, towards Paul's, all in one livery of russet cotton, 340 in number. And at Easter next, they were in blue at the Spittle, and so have continued ever since.[51]

Although is may seem like a digression to stop here to describe the distinctive clothing worn by the children of Christ's, it goes to the heart of its identity; the costume is as much a part of the foundation as the erection of the buildings. Henry Wheatley, writing in 1891, explained that "The hospital is commonly called 'The Blue Coat School', from the dress worn by the boys, which is of the same age as the foundation of the hospital."[52] The costume worn by the children of Christ's Hospital is distinctive, and contemporary students are still required to dress in the traditional uniform, with a few modifications. The revered American writer, Mark Twain, gives in *The Prince and the Pauper* a vivid description of and fashion commentary on the clothes of the orphanage/school:

> [E]ach had on the crown of his head a flat black cap about the size of a saucer, which was not useful as a covering, it being of such scanty dimensions; neither was it ornamental; from beneath it the hair fell, unparted, to the middle of the forehead, and was cropped straight around; a clerical band at the neck; a blue gown that fitted closely and hung as low as the knees or lower; full sleeves; a broad red belt; bright yellow stockings, gartered above the knees; low shoes with large metal buckles. It was a sufficiently ugly costume.[53]

The blue coats and yellow stockings are the items of apparel that have drawn the most comment. However, Christ's was not the only "blue coat" school:

> Blue Coat schools in England were particularly numerous, especially from the sixteenth century on, the best known being Christ's Hospital. . . . Why blue should have been a favourite colour for charity children is probably because in the sixteenth and seventeenth centuries it was the colour obtained from a cheap dye and worn by apprentices and servants . . . blue-dyed materials were thus originally economical and also implied a humble status.[54]

A number of schools would subsequently model their uniforms after the costumes of the children of Christ's. "At Queen Elizabeth's Hospital, Bristol, the founder, John Carr, had actually stipulated in his will in 1586 that the boys should be uniformed 'like Christ's Hospital nigh St Bartholomew's in London.'"[55] Chetham's Hospital in Manchester dressed the boys in blue, acceding to the wishes of its founder, Humphrey Chetham, who founded the school in 1656.[56] Another such school was "Colston's in Bristol, founded in 1708 by a Governor of Christ's Hospital who had its uniform copied deliberately."[57]

The yellow stockings were adopted for a specific reason. "They chose yellow stockings because they believed that the color was peculiarly inimical to lice."[58] The stockings seem to have been the subject of ridicule and were nicknamed "mustard pots." As Eleanor and Herbert Farjeon rhymed in their satire on the history of the monarchs of England in their entry on the hospital's founder:

> Edward the sixth made little noise,
> And died ere he was old;
> He loved books better than his toys,
> Or so I have been told;
> And all through him the Bluecoat Boys
> Still go in legs of gold.[59]

The girls of the orphanage/school wore costumes similar to those of the boys.

> [T]heir first gowns, in 1552, were of russet cotton and they wore a kerchief, doubtless white, which must have looked humbly medieval compared with the headdresses usual at that time. When their dresses, called 'coats', were changed to blue, the skirt was open in front in the style of the time and so exposed a yellow underskirt, the petticoat. Thus they neatly matched the boys, except that they wore an apron which was white, blue or green. The headdress at an early but uncertain date has been described as a 'coif and peak'. The coif would be a close-fitting white cap and the peak a triangular piece of white linen fastened so as to point over the forehead.[60]

With rare exceptions, it is difficult to get a grasp on the gender differences of the clothes. Sometimes the sources speak of clothes for the big boys or the small boys, but there is not one reference to clothing specifically made for the girls. Henry Machin records in his diary of 19 April 1557 that at the annual Easter sermon given at St. Mary Spital, "all the children of the hospital [were] in blue garments[,] both men children and women children. . . ."[61] There appears to be no more discrimination between the boys and girls than adopting the basic costume for female wearing.

For those who needed assurance that their charity was not being wasted, presenting well-dressed orphans before the City would serve as evidence that the City's resources were being wisely spent and justly administered. Based upon the large amount of different types of cloth annually purchased by the hospital, as recorded in the Treasurer's Account Books, it can be concluded that the youngsters received a new outfit at least once a year for Easter, if not for other church feasts as well.[62]

As already mentioned, the children were resident within the orphanage starting in November 1552, although construction and building preparations were not yet completed. The date of the onset of its operation was identified as the "first day of the erection of this house which was the 21st of November/1552."[63] Therefore, Christ's Hospital had been functioning for seven months as an orphanage and school before the official incorporation in June 1553. At that time "the young King received the Corporation at the palace, and presented them with the Charter: the children also being present at the ceremony."[64]

Therefore, the establishment of Christ's Hospital, Bridewell, and St. Thomas depended not only upon the inspiration of King Edward himself, building upon the earlier gifts of his father, but upon the Corporation of the City of London and its citizens. Edward started the process in motion, but the active cooperation of the City was needed not only to supply funds but also the personnel to oversee the proper running of these hospitals. Although Edward is credited as the founder of the hospitals, he was not the driving force behind their foundation; the citizens of London were the continuing sponsors for these charitable impulses. This was not a singular act of charity. The royal hospitals became a complex trio of institutions that demanded a great deal of time and effort by those committed to keeping them in operation.

Published in 1610, the following psalm expresses the mood and conditions surrounding Christ's foundation, and underscores the cooperation between London and the Crown.

> We orphans poor like mercy found,
> when means and friends were scant,
> our gracious God a prince did move,
> to slake and ease our want. . . .
> The groundwork of our good thus laid,
> God rais'd us patrons dear
> Whose liberal hands did still provide,
> to rid our hearts from fear.
> You citizens those patrons are;
> by you we orphans live.

Food, raiment, learning—
all we want, to us you largely give.
Bless their endeavors, Lord, we pray,
increase likewise their store,
that those in plenty may abound,
which help to feed the poor. . . .[65]

As will be shown clearly, Christ's Hospital's existed not as a warehouse for unwanted children, but as a caring place for children where they received an education. The goal of Christ's was to return these children to London society as useful and productive members of that society. The fact that Christ's Hospital still survives today as a school after four centuries is a remarkable achievement for what was, in effect, a social experiment.

2

The Structure and Administration

> So Christ's Hospital was born with, for the furtherance of learning to prevent the emergence of poverty, two petty teachers, writing and music master, and a grammar school attached. It was an institution of which the city, with justice, was particularly proud, linked with the three other hospitals in an ordered system under city management.
>
> —Joan Simon (1966)

> This is your charge, which we require of you diligently to observe. And your labours and pains herein shall be rewarded at the hands of almighty God, whom ye chiefly serve in this office. For, as the apostle saith, goodlines shall have his reward, not only in this world, but also in the world to come.
>
> —Governors of the royal hospitals (1557)

The charge just quoted was given to the treasurers of Christ's Hospital and similar charges were given to other hospital officials. It is a formal charge emphasizing a strong religious purpose. It is not possible to know if this was accepted as a personal commitment by each person taking the oath or was a mere formality; only the official records of Christ's exist, and these detail facts and decisions, not motivations or interpretations. However, based on the formal records that these men left, it is clear that the presidents, governors, officials, and staff who committed themselves to Christ's Hospital took their responsibilities seriously. Each felt his work was not only scrutinized by the others and City officials, but by God himself.

When analyzing various aspects of Christ's, the historian sometimes finds it quite modern in its operation. Christ's ultimate goal of ending poverty by nurturing children and educating them in a trade by which they could earn a decent living as adults is remarkably similar to the same goal that twentieth-century America tries to implement through a variety of social welfare programs. Christ's Hospital, nonetheless, was very much a

Tudor organization, run by an elite group of men of the City of London, and reflecting largely their attitudes and goals. The organization of Christ's was looser, less defined, more fluid, and more malleable than is possible with the strict bureaucratic structure inherent within modern companies or public institutions. This is not to say that Christ's had no guidance. The body of governors closely supervised the daily activities of the hospital; they decided policy and implemented those decisions. However, to try to lay a mantle of a modern corporation on the shoulders of the hospital obscures Christ's purpose rather than reveals the substance of its work.

It is difficult to detail precisely the makeup of the hospital personnel and their exact tasks. Unless there was a problem or a dispute, their names do not appear in hospital records. However, "job descriptions" were given to hospital officials and employees and were contained within "The Ordinances and Rules for the Governors of the Hospitals in the City of London," dated 1557. This document provides information on hospital positions and procedures. Although it is not necessarily complete, this source provides a basis for the understanding of the offices and positions within Christ's Hospital. These rules were "To be read in every of the said Hospitals at a full Court once every Quarter, either 14 days before, or after the Quarterday" as a reminder of the duties and responsibilities of those who worked for Christ's either as volunteers or as paid employees.[1] Hospital personnel fell into two basic categories: governors and paid employees. Besides sitting officially at court meetings, the governors also assumed extra duties, serving as president, treasurer, almoner, scrutener, renter, and surveyor. The hospital governors were not paid either for routine gubernatorial work or for the extra tasks some of them assumed. Christ's Hospital employed men and women for a variety of duties. These salaried employees were the clerk, the matron, the nurses, the steward, the cook, the butler, the porter, the beadles, the shoemaker, and the teaching staff.

The comptroller general and surveyor general were the officials responsible for all four hospitals. Two men, usually aldermen, were chosen annually at the general election on the basis of seniority. The records refer to "2 of the aldermen of the ancients gray-cloaks to be Governors general of all the said 4 hospitals, the senior of those twain to be Comptroller, and the other Surveyor. . . ."[2] The "generals" basically oversaw the operations of the four hospitals; their responsibilities entailed resolving disputes between hospitals or between individuals and supervising the hospitals' elections.

The comptroller general had two basic tasks. The first was to be present at the annual elections or any other meetings called to discuss matters he deemed important. After the comptroller general was informed by the treasurer of the particular hospital about the reason for calling a meeting and the agenda, the comptroller general would decide "whether he [would] be there, or not; or whether it [would] please him to appoint some other time in that behalf. . . ."[3] His second job was to receive and retain in his custody the list of the governors so that "he may perceive from time to time, who be the governors for the year ensuing for every several house."[4] The comptroller general's third responsibility was to oversee the hospitals' accounts: "That the treasurer of every house, or the clerk being thereunto appointed, do after the general audit of every house, deliver into the hands of the comptroller the just and true foot of the account of either of the houses, with the number of children and pensioner. . . ."[5]

The surveyor general's role was not as clearly defined as the comptroller general's. His most specific responsibility was to act as the comptroller's deputy. Thus, he was to attend "every general court; and the comptroller being not in town, he [was] to be warned to any such full court as shall be holden in any of the said several houses for weighty causes; and to be informed likewise by the treasurer, or the clerk by his appointment, of the causes. . . ."[6]

Although all four royal hospitals appointed these two officials to oversee their operations and they all were founded for the common purpose of helping the unfortunate poor and eliminating beggary, they clearly functioned as separate institutions because they served a different clientele. St. Thomas and St. Bart's aided the poor who were sick; Bridewell was a place of confinement for the able-bodied who had chosen begging instead of finding honest work; and Christ's primarily was a place where needy children received aid. The separate identity of each was made very clear at the general court held on 17 September 1557, when it was declared "that no Treasurer of any hospital shall meddle with the legacy in any ways that is bequeathed to another."[7] This meant that any money given to a particular hospital could not be diverted by any other laying a claim to it. This was an important policy decision, for it guaranteed to potential donors that their money would be used only at the institution that they chose to endow and would be used only for the purpose for which the donors intended. The decision also underscored the policy that each hospital's finances were to be kept separate from that of the others.

Although the hospitals were under the supervision of the Lord Mayor and aldermen, the City officials did not interfere with the operations of the hospitals unless there was a dispute or their assistance was requested. The hospitals functioned together but operated separately, each hospital being self-sufficient. The work of each hospital was different but they supplemented each other. For example, a child might be delivered to Christ's for care while the mother was taken to the workhouse at Bridewell—"A man child starved named George Dent about the age of half a year taken from the mother who was sent to Bridewell the 15th of February 1560."[8] If a person came into the care of one of the hospitals and would be better served by another, then he or she was transferred. "John Browne a vagabond in Turnagain Lane for his evil life and behavior to Bridewell, and his wife to St. Bartholomews, being deceased and a common beggar."[9] Christ's would use Bridewell as a place to put men who denied accusations of fathering illegitimate children until such time as they confessed and someone—whether they themselves, a relative, or their master (if they were apprentices)—posted a surety to support the child.

> Richard Gornell being this day was delivered out of prison who being sent to Bridewell was upon the intervention of his brother, Brian Dodme called back and the same Brian to enter into ordinary bands for keeping of the child of one Margery Sylvester which the master Richard Gornell gate with child. . . .[10]

Although maintaining completely separate fiscal accounts, it was not unheard-of for one hospital to come to the financial rescue of another. Treasurer Cage of Christ's Hospital was ordered to pay "unto John Sayer treasurer of St. Thomas Hospital to bring that house out of debt: 100Li which also was done the day above named."[11] Cooperation with each other was important to the functioning of the royal hospitals within the poor relief scheme of London. However, that did not mean there was not conflict from time to time. For example, at the court meeting on 3 May 1595, Christ's contended that St. Thomas's Hospital had somehow usurped property belonging to the orphanage and was seeking its restitution.

The head of the orphanage was the president and his authority over his hospital was such that he was to "be taken as chief ruler and governor, next unto the Lord Mayor. . . ."[12] However, the precise duties of the president are not clear. He was obliged to be present at a general court, where he represented the interests of Christ's Hospital. A general court was a meeting of presidents, governors, and officials of all the hospitals; the annual election meeting was a general court. A general court was defined as when "the greater part of the governors be assembled, that is to say, 32 at the least in number; for general causes appertaining to all the 4 houses."[13] However, he was not obliged to attend the weekly Saturday court meetings of Christ's governors held within the orphanage and did not do so unless there was something of importance on the agenda or a matter in which he held an interest was being decided. For example, in the fiscal year of 1592–93, Sir Wolstan Dixie, then president, attended no court meeting except the 21 September 1592 general court meeting for elections. Nevertheless, important decisions could not be made without his presence: "and without his person shall no weighty matters be determined or agreed upon."[14] The president had the power to call extraordinary meetings: "And his authority shall be, from time to time at his pleasure, and as to him shall seem good, to cause the number of the governors to be called together. . . ."[15] The president seems to have stayed away from the day-to-day matters of running the hospital. An important concern of the presidency seems to have involved the supervision of the governors "and to reprove and reprehend any governor in his office, if there shall appear good cause unto him."[16] If the president had been busy at the hospital on a daily basis acting as a chief executive, some notation of his activities would have been recorded by the governors. Lacking evidence to the contrary, it seems reasonable to conclude that the president of Christ's Hospital filled his position in a similar manner as the heads of present-day charitable institutions, serving, that is, as a focal point for fund raising; he also acted as a liaison between the hospital and City officials.[17]

Although the president was the nominal head, it was the body of governors who really ran Christ's Hospital. As will be shown, the administration of Christ's Hospital did not just entail the admission and discharge of children, but supervision of an extensive economic and social structure. The governors were permitted a great deal of latitude in running their hospital, and their powers were rather broadly defined as the duty to elect governors "to make and constitute good and wholesome ordinances for goodly maintenance thereof. . . ."[18] Besides the annual election and the power to make any policy that facilitated the ability to care for the poor, the governors of Christ's had other duties defined in 1556. "Ye are appointed to have the on sight order and government of Christ's hospital and of all the officers and people that in any way are lodged therein or belonging to the same. . . ."[19] The governors were also to assist the treasurer in providing "the necessary provisions of the house. . . ."[20] In essence, therefore, the governors of Christ's Hospital were charged with running the hospital well and making sure it had needed supplies. This left the governors virtually free to define their jobs themselves and, as we shall see, their assumption of duties led them in a number of directions.

The election procedure for the governors was carefully delineated. The governors held office for two years and had to be reelected biannually if they wished to continue their service; "and none to remain above 2 years, except reasonable consideration and by consent of the greatest number of the said general court."[21] Most of the governors of the hospital did serve for more than two years. The Ordinances decreed that there was to be a total of sixty-six governors to be divided evenly among the four hospitals and that fourteen of these governors were to be aldermen. The governorships were therefore broken down in the following manner: "for every house 16 persons at the least, to wit, 3 aldermen . . . and 13 commoners, whereof one shall be their Treasurer."[22]

The first step in the election process was for the governors of all four hospitals to gather together twenty days prior to election day to "nominate and put in writing the names of such number of grave citizens as by their discretion shall be thought meet to succeed in the places. . . ."[23] London was still a small enough town in the sixteenth century that it was possible for the elites to know each other and to have personal knowledge of which nominees were honest and responsible men and worthy of the challenge. The only prerequisites for nomination to a governorship were guild membership, good character, and a willingness to serve. Having completed the nominations, a general court was summoned "yearly, upon the day of St. Matthew The Apostle [21 September] . . . to be holden in Christ's Hospital, or else in some other convenient place, by the said governors or the most part of them. . . ."[24] Having made the recommendations, they had to be ratified by the Court of Aldermen.

> We the governors of the hospitals of the city of London assembled together at Christ's Hospital according to our accustomed manner and they have nominated elected and chosen aldermen [and] citizens to serve in the said hospital for the year next ensuing most humbly beseeching our lordships and brethren to ratify and confirm the same nomination and election. . . ."[25]

The administrative and fiscal year ran from Michaelmas to Michaelmas (29 September).[26] The structuring of the year in this manner corresponded with the annual elections of the City of London. Municipal elections for the sheriffs and the Lord Mayor and aldermen were held on Michaelmas. "There be in this City, according to the number of Wards 26

Aldermen, whereof yearly, on the feast day of Saint Michael the Archangel, one of them is elected to be Mayor, for the year following, to begin on the 28 of October. . . ."[27] One can conclude that such an arrangement was deliberate on the part of the governors, for they would not want to elect anyone holding the office of Lord Mayor or sheriff also to serve as governor; these City officials were too busy performing their jobs to take on any additional tasks. From the beginning, the election of governors for the royal hospitals was made part of the political ritual of Tudor London.

After nominations of citizens judged willing and able to fulfill the duties of governors, the actual election was held. The final step in the election process was to deliver the results on the day of election or the day after: "[T]he copy of the said election being confirmed by the Lord Mayor and Court of Aldermen, shall be delivered unto the comptroller. . . ."[28] Within eight days of election confirmation, the treasurers from all the hospitals were to summon their newly elected and reelected governors to their individual hospitals, where "the clerk read the general charge of every governor. . . ."[29]

Provision was made for replacement of governors who died during their term of service: "[T]he governors of the said hospital in the said house where he served, shall at the farthest within one month after his decease, at a full court, then and there elect and choose one other commoner in the place of him so deceased."[30] If the deceased were the comptroller or surveyor general, an alderman, or a hospital's treasurer, "then a General Court must be held in Christ's Hospital within ten days of his death to pick a replacement."[31]

At the general meeting in September, some of the governors were given the additional obligation of verifying the treasurer's accounts and thus were chosen auditors. After examining the treasurer's books once a year, each of the auditors would sign the account, verifying the same.

Special assignments were given to the governors as the need arose. For example, on 9 November 1597 Governors Gardner, Bates, and Langely were appointed to make an inspection of the state of repair of a room of Blackwell Hall, a property and source of income administered by the hospital. On 2 December 1560, seven governors were appointed to inspect the tenements belonging to the orphanage, especially the ones located in St. Anthony's Honeylane, St. Michael's Querne, and St. Andrew's Undershaft and to make notation of any necessary repairs.[32]

After the president and the body of governors, the most important hospital officials were the treasurers. The treasurer, who himself was also a governor, was basically responsible for paying the bills and keeping track of the hospital's income. There was no time limitation upon his tenure of office; apparently the treasurer served as long as he wished and did his job well. Christ's was fortunate in that its treasurers each served for many years: John Jackson was treasurer for twelve years, Thomas Hall for nine, William Norton for eleven, and Robert Cogan for six. The treasurer's charge was to

> receive and pay all such sums of money as by any means shall appertain or belong to the relieving and comforting of the poor children of this house and pensioners here paid; and to make a true and just account thereof within 3 months at the furthest, after the end of every year. . . .[33]

The treasurer was ordered to pay the regular bills relating to the "nursing of children, and ordinary pensions, wages, and fees" within twenty days, but extraordinary expenses needed the authorization of three governors, one of whom had to be an almoner.[34] The treasurer's job entailed supervision of all matters relating to the hospital's economy including the power

> to call before [him] all such persons or officers as have the collection or gathering of any sum or sums of money due to the said house, and to demand an account of their doing; as well of the collectors of the parishes, as also of the scrutiners, almoners, renters. . . .[35]

Within a month of acceptance of his position, the treasurer was commanded to receive "an inventory of all and all manner of goods in the said hospital. . . ."[36] He kept an annual accounting of goods while he remained in office and inspected departing hospital employees to ensure they didn't leave with the orphanage's property. Because of the need for the treasurer's presence on an almost daily basis, he was frequently the only governor on duty and as such was given authority

> to examine all such beggars, vagabonds, strumpets, or single women gotten with child . . . and them to examine, commit to prison, reprove, banish, put to labour, punish, or being diseased to admit into the hospitals. . . .[37]

Almoners—three specially appointed governors—had varied duties of inspection; they served for a year but were eligible for reappointment. The process of selection was not specified; almoners were probably chosen from governors volunteering their services. "There were also certain of the governors to be almoners and to have the on sight of this house as well that the officers should do their duties as also to see the children well governed and served and to have things necessary for them, the houses to be kept sweet. . . ."[38] The second responsibility of the almoners was to keep track of the number of children housed within and without the hospital and those people receiving pensions "for fear that you not knowing the true number, I shall exceed in burdening and charging of the house."[39] Unlike the treasurer, who was also responsible for knowing how many children the hospital cared for and the number of pensioners, the almoners were not authorized fiscal agents of Christ's, paid no bills, and did not keep financial records. In short, the almoners were general administrators, having the general daily oversight of the hospital and its employees. The following gives a brief description not only of the almoner's job but of that of some other hospital workers as well.

> Also ye shall enquire of their diet and entertainment; and of the quietness of the house; and whether every officer in his calling do his duty; as the school masters in teaching; the matron in governing the women, and keeping the provision of beds, sheets, shirts and other committed to her charge; the nurses in washing and keeping clean the children; the steward in providing victuals in due time, and at reasonable prices; the cook in wholesome dressing and clean serving of the same; the butler in dividing their proportion of bread and drink; the porter in giving of his attendance upon the safe keeping of the house; the keeper of your coal house in saving of your fuel, and keeping clean of the cloister, and all other outward parts of the house; and the clerk in writing and entering of things done and determined from time to time. . . .[40]

If any of the staff were negligent in their duties, the almoners were to warn them to improve their job performance. If the warning was not effective, then the almoners were to put the matter before the governors at a full court, where it would be decided if the offender was to be dismissed.[41] The hospital utilized the services of two governors volunteering to serve as scruteners. Like the almoners, the process for selection of this position was not delineated; the term of office was for a year, but scruteners could serve for more than one year, pending approval of their colleagues. This position entailed the scruteners to "diligently to search and enquire from time to time for all such gifts, legacies, and bequests, as have or shall be given or bequeathed to Christ's."[42] They were in charge of ensuring that any and all sums of money donated to the orphanage were actually collected and given immediately to the treasurer.[43] These fund-raisers were also obliged to keep a book that they were to "bring to the auditors of the house when the treasurer maketh up his account, to the intent the legacies by you collected may be conferred with the receipts that the treasurer shall make received of you."[44] The scruteners were also to solicit funds for the orphanage whenever possible: "[W]hen you shall happen to be in company of good virtuous and wealthy men, you shall to the best and uttermost of your wits and powers advance, commend, and set forth the order of the said hospital . . . "[45]

One governor was appointed renter. His charge was "quarterly to collect and gather for the term and space of one whole year, all these rents that shall be contained in a rental," and once collected to turn them over to the care of the treasurer.[46]The renter was also the hospital official responsible for ensuring that necessary repairs to hospital property were carried out.

Two surveyors were appointed by the hospital from the body of governors. Their job was to keep track of tenements and lands belonging to Christ's. Every March they were to report on the tenements "with the places and streets where they are, and their yearly value; with the names of the tenants; and upon the head of every tenement are be noted the term of years, if it be let out by lease, and whether the lord or tenants be bound to reparations."[47]

In addition to their specific duties, the officers of the hospital were to report abuses and to do their own job and not interfere with anyone else's work. "And you shall not make or meddle in any other man's office, but duely do your own. But if you see any thing amiss in them, you shall certify the governors thereof, that they may take order therein."[48] However, no guidance was provided to the officials to help them distinguish between interference and genuine concern over a problem.

The governors, acting either as a body or through individual governors acting as treasurers, almoners, renters, or auditors, were managers. They were to ensure that the paid staff were doing their jobs in a manner thought proper. The paid employees, those adults actually responsible for the daily care of the orphans, included a clerk, a matron, nurses, a steward, a butler, a porter, beadles, a cook, a shoemaker and the school staff. John Howes, the chronicler of Christ's early years, listed the salary for the employees in the year 1552. It can be safely assumed that wages and salaries were based upon the perceived value of labor to the employer. As such, Howes's wage schedule provides a crude idea of how important to the hospital these positions were perceived to be. The highest paid staff member was the grammar school master, John Robyson, whose annual salary was £15. The clerk, John Watson, was paid £10. Anthony Ideson, who served the hospital as cook in 1552, was paid £8 a year.[49] The steward in 1552, William Smoothing, was paid an annual fee of £6 13s. 4d., as was the butler, Thomas Mason.[50] In 1552, there were two porters, John Saepschead and John Foreskewe; they were paid £6 a piece annually for their fees.[51]

Those involved in the education of the children were paid fairly well.

> [T]he fact that Christ's Hospital was intended to be a school and not merely a nursery is clear from the beginning. One of the highest paid posts went to John Robinson, grammar school master, who received £15 a year. He had under him as "Grammar Usher" James Seamus at £10 a year, and the clerk, John Watson, in addition to his £10 a year was given another £3 6s 8d as writing master. Thomas Lowes and Thomas Cutts received £2 13s 4d a year each as "schoolmaster for music, a teacher of pricksong."[52]

The salaries of the matron and the nurses are more difficult to compare to the others because they were not only paid salaries but received additional benefits. The matron, Agnes Sexton, received as her salary £3 6s. 8d. but also received her livery (work clothes or uniforms), her lodging in the hospital, and sixteen pence a week for food.[53] Adding salary and board wages together, the matron received in money £6 16s. yearly. It is impossible to place a monetary value upon the matron's clothing allowance and rent, but salary plus benefits probably raised her compensation above the cook's £8 and possibly even up to the clerk's £10 level. Similarly, the twenty-five nurses were each paid £1 annual wage, received livery, were paid weekly 16d for a food allowance, and were also housed within the hospital.[54] The nurses received in money a total of £4 3s. 4d., and with their other benefits probably raised their compensation to the level of the stewards and butlers. According to Howes, there were additional employees, at least in 1552. Christ's also hired a barber, a tailor, two surgeons, and a coal keeper as part-time employees. The barber, John Staples, earned £2 annually. Robert Cooke, the hospital tailor, was paid a yearly fee of £2 13s. 4d. Robert Ballthroppe received the rather large annual income of £13 6s. 8d.; the other surgeon, Henry Browne, only received an annual salary of £4. The coal keeper, Trongon Charsley, was paid £2 a year, the same as the barber.[55] The highest paid salaries went to the men having special skills and education, as was the case with the schoolmaster, the clerk, and the surgeons. What is surprising is that the matron and nurses were as well paid as they were, considering that their positions required no specific skills; but this may reflect a recognition on the part of the governors that these women needed to be properly rewarded for having to be available twenty-four hours a day, seven days a week, fifty-two weeks a year.

It was the role of the clerk to keep the numerous books of the institution, and this task was not a small obligation. The range of record-keeping for the hospital is truly remarkable. It is unclear why the governors felt it was important to record any matter, large or small, touching upon Christ's. The answer may simply be that the governors were businessmen and as such were accustomed to keeping detailed records and carried that practice over into their charitable work. The records of the orphanage revolved around three areas: gubernatorial decisions, the children, and money. The clerk recorded in "a Court-book, otherwise called a Memorial-book" the business conducted at court meetings.[56] To ensure the official record properly reflected the proceedings, the clerk was ordered to "read before the breaking up or departure, that the governors may perceive thereby, whether you have entered all things to their minds or not."[57] He also kept a book on the children, "Which book shall contain the admission of any child into this house, and by what order the same was received.... Whereby the day of the month and year of their admission may appear . . ." so that the governors and staff could determine the location of the child at a glance and know "whether the same child be living and remaining in the house, or at nurse; at service, or else dead...."[58] The clerk kept track of the nursing staff in the Nurse Book, "thereby to show how many children every nurse hath, their wages weekly due for them, and a just note of the days they were delivered. . . ."[59] There was also a Pension Book wherein were kept the particulars of pensioners including their names, date of admission, and weekly stipends.[60] The clerk was responsible for keeping an annual book detailing the hospital's "collections, legacies and benevolences, box money and all other receipts and payments for the year. . . ."[61] He was also obliged to keep monthly books to chronicle

> all your receipts and payments received and paid in every month . . . board wages paid weekly to the matron, and nurses; necessaries for the household, pensioners paid in this house, with every week due to any of them: and also the like for children abroad at nurse.... And at every quarters and the fees and wages of officers. . . .[62]

Although, to ease the burden of the treasurer, the clerk was authorized to pay some bills and receive income, he had to give a monthly accounting to the treasurer of his activities. The clerk also kept a book "wherein shall be entered all debts owing to the house by composition, and therein declare their time of payment, and the manner of the bands; and also what money remain to any of the children, which was received at their admission."[63] He was also charged with keeping track of the details surrounding the hospital's ownership of land and buildings; this included "of whose gift they be; where they lie; of their butts and bounds; for what rent they go: when all their leases will be expired . . . and this book shall be entitled The Book of Lands and Tenements."[64]

Perhaps the most important aspect of the clerks' position was to be on call at all times to conduct hospital business: "to be continually attendant here in this house. . . . And all and all manner of matters what so ever at any court, or otherwise, touching the state, necessary affairs, or governance of this house. . . ."[65] Howes has recorded that the clerk of Christ's in 1552, John Watson, received £10 for his fee and livery.[66]

The job of matron mostly involved the supervision of the nursing staff, keeping the hospital clean, and keeping track of hospital supplies. The position of matron was a position of high trust and responsibility. She was obliged to live within the walls of the hospital and, as such, was available twenty-four hours a day, every day. As the highest resident official, the matron was usually called upon first to solve any problems. Even though she was only officially responsible for the female nursing staff, the matron probably also supervised to some degree the male staff, including porters and butlers, especially at those times when the governors were not available. "Your office is an office of great charge and credit. For to you is committed the governance and oversight of all the women and children within this hospital. And also to you is given authority, to command, reprove and rebuke them or any of them. . . ."[67] If any of her charges defied the matron's authority, then she was to report them to the governors, who would take further action. The matron was also responsible for seeing that the nurses washed "the children's sheets and shirts, and in keeping clean and sweet those that [were] committed to their charge; and also in the beds, sheets, coverlets, and apparel, [with keeping clean their wards and chambers] mending of such as be broken from time to time."[68] To keep the nurses busy and mindful of their chores, the matron was charged to see that the "washers and nurses of this house be always well occupied and not idle. And that their linen be wholesomely and cleanly washed; and the same first received from the keepers be (after the washing thereof) quietly delivered unto them."[69] The matron was assigned to make sure that the nurses strictly followed the procedures for the admission of children: "that no child be received by them, before the name of the same child be entered into the Ward-book; nor that any be delivered to nurse or otherwise, but that they be also entered, and to whom they are delivered, with the day and month when the same is done. . . ."[70] It also rested upon the shoulders of the matron to ensure "that the hall be kept sweet and clean; and [to] suffer none of the children to be there after their meals, except it be at service time. . . ."[71]

The matron's position entailed keeping close watch over hospital supplies. "You shall also once every quarter of the year, examine the inventory which shall be delivered unto you, of the implements of the house; as of beds, bolsters, mattresses, blankets, coverlets, sheets, pallads, shirts, hosen, and such other. . . ."[72] The matron was charged to report if any goods were "purloined, embezzled, spoiled, or otherwise consumed; and to make such lack and faults, as by you shall be espied, known unto the almoners of this house for the time being, that they may take order therein."[73]

The matron was responsible for retrieving "from the nurses in the country, when any children die their apparel."[74] And lastly, the matron was ordered to "twice or thrice in every week arise in the night, and go as well into the sick ward as also into every other ward, and there see that the children be covered in the beds, whereby they take no cold."[75]

As already stated, the matron's job was one of high trust and responsibility, and one matron, Elizabeth Cooke, widow, was fired when she betrayed that trust. On 10 November 1593, the Court of Governors decided to suspend Mistress Cooke: "ye keys of ye charges are taken from her & deliver[ed] to Master Treasurer to be disposed as he thinketh good."[76] She was accused of not being "faithful in her place," which seems to revolve around Mistress Cooke's appropriation of a child's money. Some children came into Christ's with a sum of cash that was held by hospital authorities until the child was of age. Elizabeth refused to deliver her keys and a further order was taken at the Court of Governor's meeting on 19 February 1593/94 to remove the former matron from the hospital.[77] The governors were forced to take more drastic action against Elizabeth on 6 July 1594 for her refusal to leave her lodging. The treasurer was ordered to "shut up her doors & to hang a padlock upon them."[78] Apparently that action was not effective, because the governors furthered ordered on 14 September 1594 that Elizabeth be locked out of her house and her goods confiscated and used to pay the "portion of a child in this house named Alice Richardson at ye discretion of ye governors."[79] Elizabeth Cooke's use of the child's portion forced the governors to demand on 28 September 1594 that the remaining £6 be paid off for a weekly sum after she entered a surety. That closed the episode.[80] Mistress Smothinge was dismissed from her post, but as a reward of her past services and "in consideration of her age and weakness" she was granted a pension of 2s. weekly and was given lodging within the hospital "upon her good behavior and the pleasure of the governors. . . ."[81]

Although the matron was accountable for the general well-being of the children, it fell to the nursing staff to tend directly to the physical needs of all the children, not merely to the sick. "Ye shall also carefully and diligently oversee, keep, and govern all those tender babes and younglings that shall be committed to your charge, and the same wholesomely, cleanly, and sweetly nourish and bring up."[82] The nurses were ordered to bathe their children every night and have a nightly bed check: "[S]ee that all your children before they be brought to bed, be washed and clean . . . and once every night arise, and see that the children be covered, for taking of cold."[83] In addition to tending to the children, the nurses were required to "keep [the] wards and every part thereof sweet and clean."[84] The nursing staff were also to keep themselves busy. "Ye shall also, to avoid all idleness, when your charge and care of keeping the children is past, occupy yourselves in spinning, sewing, mending of sheets and shirts, or some other virtuous exercise. . . ."[85] In more general terms, the nurses were told, "Your charge is faithfully and truly to serve in this house, to obey the matron thereof. Ye shall also fly and eschew all railing, scolding, swearing and drunkenness. Ye shall in your behavior and doings be virtuous loving and diligent."[86] Failure to do their work properly and observe the rules would result in any "correction and punishment that shall be thought meet, by the discretion of the governors, but also to be expulsed and banished [from] this house forever."[87]

Christ's Hospital also employed a steward whose job was basically to supply the necessary provisions. "Your office shall be to provide all such necessary victuals . . . as of butter, cheese, fish, wood, coal, etc. . . . as shall be assigned from time to time by the treasurer or almoners of the house, to the use of the poor. . . ."[88] He had the responsibility to "deliver the due proportion appointed for every meal" unto the cook. "And this shall you daily do in the presence of the matron or one of the almoners of the house."[89] The steward received the following stern warning: "You shall not embezzle or convey any manner of victuals, either to your own use, or to the use of any person, other than to the use of this house as aforesaid; upon pain to be deprived of the house and lose your office for ever."[90] The butler's duty was to receive the provisions for the hospital. "Your office shall be to receive of the baker and brewer, such bread and drink, as shall from time to time be appointed by the governors of this house, for the use of the poor."[91] Ensuring the proper service of food was also his responsibility. "And the same to deliver again to the use of the poor at every meal; after such manner and proportion, as shall be appointed you by the treasurer or almoners of that house."[92] They were additionally instructed to "have no manner of fees, but your ordinary wages."[93]

The porter was concerned with the security of Christ's and keeping close watch over those entering or leaving the premises. "You shall be attendant diligently and carefully in looking to the gates. . . ."[94] His main chore was to close the gates at nightfall "and see [the children] shut in at a due hour, and after they be shut in, to be circumspect whom you let in and out."[95] Since the time of nightfall varied with the season, the porter received instruction on when to close the gate:

> after the hour of nine of the clock in the winter season, not to open the gates in any wise, except on a very great occasion. And in summer season, you shall keep the gates open no longer than nine of the clock; and you shall, after they be shut in, neither let any in nor out after ten of the clock at the furthest.[96]

On 4 December 1560, Robert Cook, haberdasher, and the hospital's tailor, was appointed to be both porter and butler of Christ's. "[T]o whom was granted for his wages yearly 3Li and daily in bread. 2d and in beef daily 2lb. and in beer daily one gallon. with the like allowance for the fish day."[97] This appointment was in reaction to the earlier dismissal of Trinian Carsley, porter and keeper of the wood and coal, and William Beane, butler, who were dismissed on 21 October 1560 for unstated reasons. It was thereby resolved that one man would fill both positions.[98]

The beadles were responsible, in general, for keeping the peace within the twenty-six wards of the City of London. They were always obliged to "carry your tipstaffs in your hands, and wear your blue liveries. . . ."[99] The beadles were ordered to visit daily "all such wards as [were] appointed for your walk; and shall cleanse all the same wards from beggars and other idle people; and the same people so found to drive away, or to carry to Bridewell."[100] If met with resistance "by way of the said vagrants and evil persons, you shall call for aid to every constable next adjoining to assist you."[101] If there was a death within their jurisdiction, the beadles received the following instruction: "[G]ive your attendance at the houses of them so deceased; and . . . see that no rogues or idle persons resort thither to trouble the street."[102]

In addition, they were required "to attend at this hospital, upon the treasurer and governors of the same hospital; and to be ready and willing to execute such business as the said treasurer and governors or any of them shall command you."[103] The beadle's job was also "according to the old custom, give . . . attendance upon the lord mayor at the Guildhall, the Sessions house and Bridewell; and there perform your office as you are commanded. . . ."[104] Every beadle was ordered "every Sunday, with the rest of the beadles of the other houses, shall give your attendance at Paul's Cross at the sermon time; to visit all the streets and lanes adjoining, and there to apprehend all such vagrant and idle persons, as shall be there found . . . and to carry them, as well men, as women and children, to Bridewell. . . ."[105] The beadles were subject to annual appointment at the election of governors and others in September. "[I]f any of them be faulty, . . . he or they may be rebuked or dismissed, at the discretion of the said court," and ordered to turn over their staves.[106] However, if a beadle died in office, then the Court of Governors appointed a replacement, as was the case with John Pearce, who assumed a job as beadle on 22 January 1592/93 in "the place of William Dukinsons late beadle." Pearce was "to continue in the same during the pleasure of the Governors."[107]

The cook's sphere within the hospital went beyond practicing the culinary arts. The first chore of the cook was the supervision of meat preparation. "Your office is to dress such meat as shall be delivered unto you by the steward, to the use of the poor, wholesomely and cleanly."[108] The cook was ordered to "receive no meat of the said steward, but in presence of the matron of the house, or of one of the almoners."[109] All the received meat was to be entered into a book that was to be "conferred with the steward's book; and your said book shall be subscribed, or signed by the matron or almoners . . . present. And the same steward [was] to have his allowance, according to the book so subscribed and not otherwise."[110] An additional order was given to the cook forbidding any "manner of fee profit or other commodity, as tallow, ashes or any other, but only your wages and livery."[111]

Christ's Hospital even had a resident shoemaker who supplied the leather for shoes. However, his function also involved teaching the children his craft.[112]

Hospital officers and staff were expected to perform their duties earnestly and honestly. When corruption was discovered, the governors launched an investigation. Such was the case with the clerk of Christ's, Richard Wilson, who held that position from 1585 until 1591. Wilson was accused of deceitfulness and "abusing of the Accounts" after a routine audit by William Norton, then the treasurer, and the governors in November of 1593. This was a serious affair, because the clerk was not only in charge of keeping records of all hospital business but was one of two authorized agents for the receipt of money, the other being the treasurer. Basically, the former clerk was charged with stealing. As the governors phrased it,

> [H]e deceived ye hospital of great sums of money and for that this court think it convenient that this falsehood be discovered & laid open for ye satisfying of ye mayor & aldermen & other worshipful citizens of this city into whose hearers the rumor of the said Wilson's deceit is come. . . .[113]

On 10 November 1593, Richard Wright, the hospital's solicitor, was ordered to investigate the matter further and assess the financial damage done to the orphanage. This disturbing affair ended on 14 November 1593 when the said Wilson confessed to all charges at a governors' meeting, promising full cooperation and to make complete restitution of all monies taken. As a token of his good faith, he made "a gift of all his goods & promising to be ready at al times to satisfy ye governors. . . ."[114]

As we have seen, the duties of most hospital officers and staff were laid out in the Ordinances, but the particular responsibilities of the most visible group of people associated with Christ's, the governors themselves, were not defined. Having already discussed the election procedure for the governors and the rather broad definition of their responsibilities, the question still needs to be answered, What exactly did the governors do when they were serving in their capacities as ordinary governors, not as almoners or in other positions? Their main responsibility was to appear at the weekly Saturday court meeting, where the major business of Christ's Hospital was conducted. A carefully kept record of those meetings exists in three volumes for the years 1552–98 in the manuscript entitled "Minutes of the Court of Governors." The governors dealt with all manner of matters affecting the hospital, including the admission and dismissal of children, the granting of pensions, ensuring adequate supplies of food and other necessities, and supervising Christ's staff and officers. A study of their records reveals that the governors had three main concerns besides the admission and care of children. These were to maintain income, to reduce beggary, and to locate fathers of illegitimate children and force them to pay for their children's care.

Judging by the entries in the Minutes, there were two areas of the hospital's income-generating power that attracted a good deal of the governors' energies: regulation of hospital property and Blackwell Hall. The management of their properties in a rapidly expanding London was a complicated business. Rents accounted for 8.6 percent of total income (see chapter 3). The role of Christ's Hospital as a landlord and its interaction with London society is a subject beyond the scope of this book and needs further investigation. The renting and maintenance of property could only be done by the Court of Governors. Hence the proviso "That no sale of land, timber or wood; lease, alienation, building or reparation be determined or done, of lands or tenements. . . ."[115] Hospital property was rented according to a fairly standard formula, and the following is a typical lease agreement:. "[T]hat is ordered that one John Stapleford shall have a lease of a tenement in kinstreet Westminster at 5Li rent per annum and 60 Li fine vz. 20Li in hand and 20Li at year's end."[116] Although the length of time that this lease was to be in effect was not specified in this example, usually leases were awarded for the period of twenty-one years.[117] The hospital not only charged £5 annual rent but a £60 fine, as a down payment. It should also be noted that the fine was not required to be paid all at once but according to the following schedule: £20 immediately, £20 at the end of the 1591–92 fiscal year, and the last £20 to be paid at the end of the second year. Sometimes, leases were granted on a conditional basis. A carpenter by the name of Thomas Grigson was granted a lease for forty years at the cost of an annual rent of £2 for a garden and "for the gate in the town ditch called the back gate. . . ." This lease was granted upon condition that the said Grigson "build a new house of good and strong timber. . . ."[118] After a lease was granted there was a set procedure for the requisite paperwork.

> [A]ll the same leases be drawn in paper by a scrivenor, one of the governors of the said hospital before they be engrossed . . . and the clerk of the said hospital to engross them, and to procure the sealing of all such leases before the Lord Mayor and Court of Aldermen in the chamber of London, where the common seal of the hospital doth remain.[119]

The management of the properties owned by Christ's necessitated careful regulation by the governors. In addition to granting leases, the governors were busy managing all the details that come with being a landlord. One of their tenants, Thomas Haselwood, had made a hole in a wall so that he could "cast out his dung . . . into a garden room there (for the which he paith 20s. yearly)."[120]

Like modern landlords, Christ's Hospital was responsible for repairs to its buildings. On occasion, the orphanage neglected to carry out necessary repairs due to the lack of funds, as was the case with a property on New Fish Street. It had been so neglected that on 6 May 1570, the governors decided to dismantle the old building and build a new structure. It was further decided to let Mr. Goffe, who held the lease on that property, to continue with the original lease arrangement.[121]

The governors also had the administration over Blackwell Hall, a depot for cloth in London, and the income generated from this endeavor accounted for over one-fourth of the annual income for the hospital. When the amount of money coming into the orphanage from Blackwell Hall started dropping off dramatically in the 1590s, due to a severe slump in the wool trade, the governors expressed alarm. In fact, starting in 1593, there was almost no governors' court meeting when the subject of Blackwell Hall was not discussed in some fashion. How to increase revenue and how to improve operating efficiency were of special concern (see chapter 3 for more information on Blackwell's revenue problems).

As mentioned, the governors also spent a lot of time and energy upon locating and forcing fathers to pay for their illegitimate children rather than leaving them to the charity of the citizens of London. Unmarried mothers needed to go before the governors and name the father. More often than not, the governors believed the women and the men had to prove their innocence; the women didn't have to prove the men guilty. It was probably one of the few instances in Western culture in which women were given the benefit of the doubt in a legal conflict.

To a certain degree, the governors' procedure was self-serving, because if a man was found by them to be the father of a bastard and forced to pay "child support" or marry the mother, then the City was spared the cost of maintaining that child. An interest in enforcing a strict standard of morality and thereby ensuring the status quo worked together with the more pragmatic interest in money. The fact is that throughout the years of its operation Christ's hospital was operating on the verge of insolvency, and every penny and shilling made a difference to the survival of the orphanage.

Not every accused man was found guilty of fathering the child in question. For example, Hugh Robertson was alleged by Alice Harcote of seducing her and getting her with child "upon Bartholomew Day in the fore noon. . . ."[122] When Robertson produced neighbors who claimed that he was with them on the day and time in question, the charges were dropped.

There was a set procedure for examining the mothers of illegitimate children.

> And that two governors or more, whereof the treasurer to be one . . . shall also at any time examine all single women or others being brought into this house with child; and cause the parties whom they accuse to be sent for before them; and upon his or their confession, to cause him or them to enter into bands with sureties to the mayor and commonality, to see the same child kept from the charge of this city and hospitals; and to see the woman provided for, from that time until she be delivered and churched; with such other covenants as the case shall require. And if the said parties do not confess the fact, and the same by all presumptions likely to be true, they shall be committed to ward, there to remain until further trial may be had thereof; or else put in sureties to answer this court from time to time, until the truth may be known.[123]

The women who came before the court to identify the father of their children supplied detailed information on the circumstances surrounding their seduction.

> Alice Bruster servant with William Sayuell Budgemaker dwelling in Paul's church yard declared that her said Master gate her with child and she saith that he promised her marriage and abused her half a dozen times in the Shop & other places & he said if his wife died he would. . . .[124]

That same day, Sayvell was called before the court, where he denied the charge of fathering Alice's child and making a proposal of marriage. At the next regular court day, 26 November 1569, the accused William Sayvell still declared his innocence and that he "never had to do with Alice Bruste. . . ."[125] At the same court, Alice maintained that three witnesses, Mistress Benlew, Goodwife Robinson, and Mistress Claiden, heard William Sayvell say to them that if Alice "would have keep the matter secret that he would have allowed to her 2s or forty pence a week. . . ."[126] All these five people were ordered to appear at the next court. At the governors' court on 10 December 1569, Sayvell finally admitted the fact and promised "to keep her the time she liethe in childbed and further to give her 20£ . . . or else marry her."[127]

Accused fathers were required to post a bond to insure their appearance on court days. For example, Hugh Robertson was required to give a surety of £10 on 12 August 1570. That was a hefty sum of money. Ten pounds was more than many people paid for their yearly rent or earned in annual wages.[128] In addition, some men were incarcerated either in Bridewell or in the hospital's stockhouse until either confessing the deed or posting a surety. Locking up these men did tend to elicit a confession rather quickly from them. For example, at the 14 October 1570 meeting of the Court of Governors, Margaret Cale claimed that Henry Carie had "gotten her with child the first time that he abused her . . . about 3 weeks before Easter last . . . and again abused her 14 days after Easter. . . ."[129] Carie was examined at the same Court, denied the charge, and was confined in the hospital's stockhouse until he could post a surety. Although the governors generally believed the women, especially when they could provide details on the time and place of the sexual activity, having a witness did lend extra credibility to their cases. Cicely Somerset's witness said that around Christmas 1571 she had observed that Richard Ryley, a gardener from Southwork, "in the night time came to the windmill in St. George's field with a great dog lead in his hand and fetched out . . . Cecily . . . after whom she looked out and saw the same Ryley abuse her body in a pit. . . ."[130] Richard was ordered to post bond for the purpose of supporting the child.

A promise of marriage used as part of a seduction was looked upon most gravely by the governors, and with good reason. The Catholic Church's definition of a valid marriage was still accepted in Tudor England. There were two components necessary for a legal marriage: free consent, which involved a promise or agreement to accept each other as husband and wife, and sexual intercourse. Therefore, if a man promised marriage in order to seduce a girl and then they had intercourse, this was construed to be a valid marriage, even without some kind of public nuptial or wedding ceremony.[131] Rachel Griffin came to court in January or early February in 1571/72 claiming that Henry Norrison got her with child, having abused "her on midsummer [24 June] evening in the kitchen and diverse times before that and that he promised her marriage. . . ."[132] The record of this matter is a bit garbled, but it appears that a Robert Wheatly also had had sexual relations with Rachel. With paternity uncertain, the court ordered both Wheatley and Norrison to pay her an allowance during her pregnancy and to pay her child support. What is interesting about this case is that neither man could evade his responsibility by claiming that another could also be held liable.

Other expectant fathers were required to pay child support and support until the child was born. James Aborrow appeared at a court on 17 February 1570/71 with his master, Thomas Newam, brewer, and made the following arrangement with Katherine Ouerton: "to give her 6d weekly until she be brought abed and then during her laying on childbed to allow her 20s and then to take away. . . ."[133] Masters were financially liable for the cost of their servant's illegitimate children; they were responsible for the sexual activity of everyone in their household, in the same way as a parent was answerable for the cost of raising a child until it reached the legal age of maturity.

Illegitimacy was a stain not only upon the child but upon the mother. Men in sixteenth-century London were held accountable for their sexual activity, forced to confess before town officials, and forced to pay money for the care of their children; the City would not permit men to seduce women, get them pregnant, and then abandon them to public charity. What is particularly interesting in the many dozens of cases recorded in the Book of Minutes of the Court of Governors is that the women were not only believed but were treated with respect. The governors hurled no invectives against the women; they were not treated as whores or morally deficient people. Part of this treatment may have resulted from the fact that it was sometimes difficult to tell from the evidence whether the sexual activity was from seduction or outright rape. This was especially so in the cases where masters had abused their servants or apprentices. This meant breaking a fundamental bond of trust and responsibility. Masters were expected to function as fathers to their charges. In contrast to the prevailing attitude of Western society that women are to blame for the sexual indiscretions of men, especially rape, the governors seemed to hold the men responsible for seducing these women.

Although Christ's tended to the needs of abandoned, sick, disabled, or just plain poor children, the governors also felt a strong impetus to curb the scourge that threatened the security of their City, beggary. Any activity or policy that tended to prevent begging was taken up by the governors, although it may seem not to have much to do with the care of children. This could involve, for instance, pensioning those groups of people, such as disabled soldiers and the elderly, who were often destitute and forced to beg. Tudor Englishmen wanted to draw a sharp distinction between those who by reason of age or physical disability and were unable to work, and therefore could be given help, and the able-bodied poor who were too lazy to work and therefore should be forced to support themselves and their families.

On 7 December 1556, the governors of Christ's found it necessary to post citizen guards at the gates of the City to prevent beggars from entering.

> An order also taken for the keeping of the ten ports or gates of this city by ten honest citizens to avoid all such as might lay children in the streets or any vagabond, beggar or other idle person which daily frequenteth to the same, and to any of the same, is grant yearly . . . for the keeping of the same. . . .[134]

The hospital's governors, the following year, felt compelled to take further action to make it easy to identify those receiving public assistance and to therefore make it harder to defraud the City.

> And it was also devised and agreed that certain badges of lead should be made that any poor and pensioner with in the city should wear upon their breast to be known by, and that in any parish . . . some other honest person should be appointed who should attend daily upon their own parish to kept out from begging within the same all foreign and strange beggars. . . .[135]

At a general court meeting on 12 March 1568/69, the governors of all four hospitals agreed to force vagabonds to clean the sewers and ditches, a very nasty job indeed and an early example of trying to force criminals into performing socially useful work. By this time, begging was no longer perceived as an unavoidable response of poor people to desperate circumstances, but was considered a criminal act. Since beggars were now criminals it was acceptable to treat them in harsh ways and to mark them by placing "a collar of iron about the necks. . . ."[136]

In reviewing the administrative structure of Christ's Hospital, it needs to be stressed again that the orphanage was run by two types of people: officers, who were also governors, and salaried employees. The hospital was run according to set procedures to insure its efficient operation. Although the duties of the hospital staff were carefully defined, the duties of the body of governors were not specifically laid out. It was probably felt that any attempt to define their duties would hamper the effectiveness of the governorships. The governors were allowed a great latitude to interpret their roles. In fact, they seemed to wield a great deal of power. This assumption of power by the governors is not surprising; these were the same men who ran the political and financial institutions of London. At times, the Court of Governors functioned almost as a law court, as we have seen with bastards' fathers. Any action that reduced costs or alleviated any aspect of poverty was acceptable, even if that sometimes meant the extension of gubernatorial authority beyond tending to the needs of the children under their care.

Having discussed the administrative structure of Christ's Hospital and the personnel involved with operating the orphanage, a discussion of its complex fiscal structure is in order and will take up the next two chapters.

Table 1. Revenues and Expenditures (1552–98)

Year	Annuity	Bay Hall	Benevolences	Blackwell Credits	Blackwell Debits	Blackwell Income
1552	na	na	na	na	na	na
1553	14.3917	na	na	na		na
1554	na	na	43.9800	na	na	na
1555	10.8000	na	540.2009	0.6667	na	0.6667
1556	37.5500	na	16.5001	na	na	na
1557	na	na	37.4400	391.8291	na	391.8291
1558	na	na	na	na	na	na
1559	na	na	19.7833	na	na	na
1560	na	na	na	na	na	na
1561	na	na	63.6250	na	na	na
1562	8.4000	na	na	1372.7329	3.4000	1369.3329
1563	13.2000	na	32.3083	157.9500	60.7333	97.1967
1564	na	na	26.4958	660.3457	3.4000	656.9457
1565	na	na	36.2250	761.1499	8.4000	752.7499
1566	6.6000	na	259.1001	723.0957	8.4000	714.6957
1567	5.4250	na	19.6750	802.7542	68.4000	734.3542
1568	na	na	27.3500	644.7332	68.4000	576.3332
1569	12.1583	na	39.6104	611.4165	68.4000	543.0165
1570	1.2167	na	25.0750	612.5708	68.4000	544.1708
1571	7.3667	na	46.1167	659.3416	68.0334	591.3082
1572	14.1750	na	45.5541	655.8206	67.6667	588.1539
1573	8.6583	na	44.2917	782.1809	37.3667	744.8142
1574	10.0500	na	86.0542	908.9370	9.1334	899.8036
1575	5.4000	28.5292	165.1125	827.9998	2.6667	825.3331
1576	6.7302	50.6167	59.3417	944.7827	4.1334	940.6493
1577	8.1167	84.6167	128.0583	1070.7952	9.0667	1061.7285
1578	8.0625	80.5667	68.2833	1012.5767	41.0667	971.5100
1579	12.9000	98.0750	151.0167	1069.6499	11.4792	1058.1707
1580	9.6750	186.0647	68.3083	1067.9414	46.4792	1021.4622
1581	11.8084	62.1458	67.4166	1094.3330	47.4000	1046.9330
1582	12.2604	94.9792	48.1667	1150.5850	11.1083	1139.4767
1583	10.6500	47.4375	58.4417	1099.4727	12.8125	1086.6602
1584	11.8562	108.9688	14.3833	1103.6707	47.4000	1056.2707
1585	8.4000	122.6062	125.8917	1182.7827	81.7457	1101.0370
1586	27.9125	57.9917	29.8083	1064.1079	104.4790	959.6289
1587	32.8250	63.8042	54.6646	867.9956	107.6458	760.3498
1588	21.5584	49.6167	29.2500	797.8511	110.4125	687.4386
1589	13.0417	35.3750	61.3500	772.7769	182.7957	589.9810
1590	23.0750	107.2042	23.8583	778.3474	110.4125	667.9349
1591	34.6874	11.3542	75.1917	738.7622	112.0625	626.6997
1592	28.8500	98.4104	102.3375	804.3372	60.3125	744.0247
1593	na	na	na	na	na	na
1594	18.8500	9.2917	17.1917	542.8892	158.1542	384.7350
1595	53.5416	na	49.1125	778.5723	132.8125	644.7598
1596	37.5792	77.8083	16.5667	757.9868	86.8292	671.1576
1597	79.7876	na	28.9792	854.0371	85.0635	768.9736
1598	44.4665	na	78.8875	872.6729	103.5664	769.1065
Min	1.2167	9.2917	14.3833	0.6667	2.6667	0.6667
Max	79.7876	186.0647	540.2009	1372.7329	182.7957	1369.3329
Avg	18.6674	73.7731	71.4879	815.8013	61.3900	757.6156
St Dev	15.9893	40.6510	88.1125	266.0341	46.4807	274.8595

Money is calculated in English pounds; *na* = data not available or missing data.

Table 1. *(continued)*

Year	Boxes	Building Staff	Burial	Butter	Carmen	Cheese
1552	8.0646	na	na	na		na
1553	84.4332	220.5500	na	9.4417	na	na
1554	46.7698	38.1167	na	na	na	na
1555	84.9657	15.2208	na	10.8417	na	na
1556	9.2458	28.6042	na	57.7001	na	na
1557	28.9980	na	na	na	na	na
1558	16.7916	na	na	na	na	na
1559	27.2500	na	na	na	na	4.8333
1560	na	na	na	na	na	na
1561	40.3416	na	na	na	na	1.3000
1562	na	na	na	19.8000	na	2.4500
1563	37.0531	14.9000	na	37.0000	na	2.9500
1564	27.1230	37.6458	na	na	na	3.3500
1565	29.4667	3.6666	na	44.8792	na	7.9667
1566	35.2979	12.6333	na	11.7500	na	5.6417
1567	32.5000	6.5333	na	14.5500	na	8.4833
1568	29.6552	12.0500	na	34.6833	na	3.9333
1569	36.7608	41.9625	na	23.2208	na	5.9333
1570	31.8354	0.2000	na	22.5083	na	4.7500
1571	32.6250	7.0750	13.0000	28.6000	na	4.7500
1572	33.2833	127.9374	na	39.4750	na	4.4167
1573	31.0510	5.7125	na	42.1000	na	4.2667
1574	38.8375	na	na	28.2917	na	4.9167
1575	29.7271	8.0667	na	19.8625	na	5.9167
1576	39.3760	25.2000	na	46.1833	na	na
1577	33.9250	28.6104	na	30.4167	na	12.7667
1578	36.4385	40.3833	24.0333	23.4458	na	7.6667
1579	32.3823	35.1834	na	42.2271	na	4.9167
1580	44.0010	18.6416	50.8333	40.2604	na	15.9333
1581	40.4188	3.0875	45.0833	34.5499	na	16.7000
1582	44.2652	15.5209	38.0083	40.0042	na	20.7000
1583	37.3729	5.8000	56.9000	25.9125	150.0000	31.6500
1584	41.9375	37.3667	78.6000	52.3062	150.3917	24.0000
1585	44.4833	0.5000	127.6667	53.6958	206.1292	21.5167
1586	42.1198	6.6228	94.1583	33.2000	142.5292	22.2167
1587	39.8010	na	112.0833	51.7937	145.0583	29.4167
1588	48.5758	na	107.7667	44.5125	112.6417	32.9167
1589	na	2.2583	74.0292	57.8146	173.9958	25.2667
1590	39.6948	na	94.8200	48.5250	175.7667	26.1000
1591	39.6908	na	89.3333	64.5479	161.0750	67.0834
1592	41.8594	0.2187	130.4917	52.9104	184.3917	47.7500
1593	33.7958	na	na	24.2000	na	na
1594	na	na	58.6000	24.2000	275.1748	61.7583
1595	34.9802	0.1417	117.9500	49.9750	189.9125	87.4750
1596	36.5781	na	103.3333	28.0500	199.4792	98.6750
1597	33.9448	1.6500	193.8167	65.4917	217.2208	118.5500
1598	34.4427	na	122.3333	32.6500	223.7417	156.3917
Min	8.0646	0.1417	13.0000	9.4417	112.6417	1.3000
Max	84.9657	220.5500	193.8167	65.4917	275.1748	156.3917
Avg	37.0270	25.8729	86.6420	36.1943	180.5006	27.1705
St Dev	13.3663	42.9074	42.1078	14.7621	39.0588	35.4895

Table 1. *(continued)*

Year	Cloth	Coal	Collection	Fish	Food	Fuel
1552	na	na	na	na	na	na
1553	70.7937	123.5333	1929.4487	15.6583	494.1633	136.3999
1554	65.3619	69.3667	1895.6238	na	503.1292	98.5373
1555	67.1674	36.8167	1824.7415	0.6625	1010.8013	88.3750
1556	15.0480	136.9896	1700.7683	10.2355	873.1584	162.8771
1557	na	na	1013.2473	4.5000	122.5188	na
1558	na	3.3000	4.5667	na	na	3.3000
1559	na	na	na	na	na	na
1560	na	na	na	na	na	na
1561	na	na	266.9165	na	na	na
1562	26.0541	23.5833	838.2639	na	61.3000	49.0333
1563	99.0250	27.6000	1055.4299	na	85.8000	51.5750
1564	102.2082	21.0000	856.9812	na	36.8833	42.9000
1565	54.4645	22.9542	1754.8416	na	63.1042	45.6709
1566	212.6710	23.1667	na	na	59.4666	44.4334
1567	133.9187	23.5000	646.1853	na	84.2750	42.8333
1568	163.2375	19.0000	628.8479	na	106.2833	40.3333
1569	149.7041	23.0333	686.2646	na	43.7791	47.0416
1570	129.7293	20.8333	572.0500	na	58.5249	42.7000
1571	134.1749	27.0000	605.2083	na	86.6833	49.5000
1572	125.8959	27.3250	na	na	111.5290	49.3250
1573	214.9747	42.3459	999.5791	na	96.9749	66.6709
1574	116.0561	43.6000	22.7750	na	78.8416	65.6000
1575	195.5571	35.9833	1284.7146	na	64.8625	58.6500
1576	149.6272	28.4417	1378.9602	1.4834	116.5801	51.1084
1577	231.5478	30.8416	1019.4167	2.6000	175.0334	55.1666
1578	274.0061	31.7584	939.8457	1.4750	197.4165	56.0751
1579	247.8542	33.1000	873.2041	104.0000	403.7764	33.1000
1580	272.0620	34.6000	793.5500	1.1250	230.5728	57.6000
1581	385.4929	40.1708	668.9834	0.9500	235.2540	66.5625
1582	187.3561	37.9583	731.1416	na	259.0977	60.6250
1583	467.0315	41.7500	734.2542	na	296.9871	65.0833
1584	262.7405	17.1000	835.4082	na	277.6870	41.1000
1585	308.7974	60.3708	740.3958	na	298.3455	86.5540
1586	281.5454	37.7500	623.0979	na	771.1360	72.4667
1587	241.7978	20.1667	1322.9019	na	456.0510	46.5333
1588	258.2683	40.7167	1186.8999	na	442.0327	60.2209
1589	309.1660	35.5750	1256.1704	na	344.9136	59.7501
1590	230.1250	51.0500	624.5125	na	459.2571	69.7167
1591	229.6500	38.4958	1106.6707	na	499.7419	56.4958
1592	282.9307	40.5000	598.5332	na	310.2598	53.1667
1593	na	na	na	na	51.8124	na
1594	245.0687	48.6500	1394.8726	6.2500	244.4250	48.6500
1595	329.5369	46.8000	1111.2603	na	464.6553	65.6166
1596	283.8599	56.5000	1085.5747	7.0000	666.2759	73.9000
1597	315.0620	53.1667	1047.1853	na	915.1306	62.1667
1598	257.4041	52.3084	652.2498	na	580.6826	62.3834
Min	15.0480	3.3000	4.5667	0.6625	36.8833	3.3000
Max	467.0315	136.9896	1929.4487	104.0000	1010.8013	162.8771
Avg	203.1743	39.7244	958.8181	12.9950	303.3144	60.7268
St Dev	100.1023	24.3261	446.2466	27.7812	256.4886	25.7185

Table 1. *(continued)*

Year	Legacies	Legacies Adjusted	Legal	Meat	Milk	Miscellaneous Payments
1552	na	na	na	na	na	na
1553	na	na	6.0000	18.4417	17.6605	138.4393
1554	259.0200	212.3600	na	6.0000	46.7230	73.6957
1555	374.0005	174.0005	0.5750	99.7294	20.1333	581.6448
1556	87.3020	237.3020	5.7250	174.8416	8.1500	571.3684
1557	228.3957	88.3957	na	3.9375	na	173.5313
1558	na	na	na	na	na	25.0000
1559	221.0000	141.0000	na	na	na	na
1560	na	na	na	na	na	na
1561	119.1000	na	na	na	na	na
1562	6.7500	75.8500	na	na	na	422.9287
1563	62.6000	62.6000	na	na	na	0.9583
1564	190.4834	90.4834	na	na	na	15.0208
1565	237.7667	197.7667	na	na	na	35.5792
1566	170.2667	170.2667	na	na	na	12.8125
1567	152.9333	152.9333	na	na	na	19.5249
1568	30.4125	30.4125	na	na	na	78.2708
1569	241.6167	41.6167	na	na	na	140.7749
1570	76.9667	76.9667	na	na	na	40.9332
1571	145.0333	105.0333	na	na	na	27.5999
1572	168.0500	168.0500	na	na	na	48.3957
1573	58.3667	58.3667	na	na	na	51.6001
1574	128.7041	128.7041	na	na	na	150.9854
1575	154.1167	154.1167	1.5000	na	na	140.1540
1576	378.0208	178.0208	0.5000	na	na	129.6041
1577	332.6667	132.6667	2.0000	na	na	230.1871
1578	583.4829	193.4829	9.5000	na	na	127.1832
1579	244.1958	104.1958	4.5000	na	na	237.6904
1580	103.1667	103.1667	1.0000	na	na	234.5156
1581	290.5249	183.9067	7.8750	na	na	360.6941
1582	84.8333	84.8333	10.0000	na	na	262.4954
1583	324.7000	224.7000	66.8250	na	na	586.4268
1584	144.6700	144.6700	19.9583	na	na	69.4583
1585	624.5979	124.5979	30.9083	na	na	1161.3604
1586	438.9998	90.3333	23.7500	21.1417	na	184.1291
1587	268.6667	268.6665	92.8917	na	na	202.0999
1588	309.3333	159.3333	26.6667	na	na	606.6062
1589	313.4998	173.4998	na	na	na	96.7207
1590	182.0000	142.0000	93.1667	na	na	207.1363
1591	293.8665	293.8665	36.6667	na	na	244.2334
1592	252.5000	212.5000	26.6667	na	na	563.4331
1593	na	na	na	na	na	na
1594	211.9583	111.9583	18.8333	na	na	92.5416
1595	210.4667	170.4667	3.0000	na	na	85.7249
1596	93.5000	93.5000	16.4250	119.8917	na	980.4871
1597	393.0000	193.0000	32.2166	188.3968	na	853.9707
1598	487.6665	271.3333	23.3333	108.9989	na	44.8834
Min	6.7500	30.4125	0.5000	3.9375	8.1500	0.9583
Max	624.5979	293.8665	93.1667	188.3968	46.7230	1161.3604
Avg	230.4572	146.8518	22.4193	82.3755	23.1667	245.4952
St Dev	138.9797	62.6701	25.6579	68.3380	14.3171	272.5609

Table 1. *(continued)*

Year	Necessaries	Nursing	Pensions	Rents	Spirits	Staff
1552	na	na	na	na	na	na
1553	na	144.7536	18	83	18	244
1554	81.7909	309.0151	869	21	53	245
1555	155.8081	520.8762	67	136	81	252
1556	232.7684	630.0078	95	37	66	182
1557	85.3762	153.3335	29	na	1	41
1558	368.6941	290.7612	66	na	na	121
1559	na	na	na	18	na	na
1560	na	na	na	na	na	na
1561	109.8281	95.2874	37	na	na	8
1562	470.4734	357.7578	161	16	33	58
1563	532.0598	339.4624	155	59	36	121
1564	459.7703	356.5327	136	37	37	176
1565	446.8015	377.3164	116	26	18	92
1566	467.5474	366.8662	105	na	33	221
1567	414.0476	390.9658	117	62	64	107
1568	440.8186	407.3997	108	66	72	164
1569	487.6790	390.3164	101	64	8	236
1570	463.3569	382.8997	97	67	35	161
1571	516.0601	309.6414	93	68	51	161
1572	588.1890	294.5083	78	73	48	133
1573	695.2910	368.4082	292	69	46	173
1574	554.6577	542.1406	326	155	41	167
1575	605.9766	633.1741	339	109	40	132
1576	578.6118	200.7708	307	122	62	234
1577	557.0017	608.3452	311	188	61	178
1578	550.4119	618.1531	309	261	62	204
1579	415.9722	563.6411	216	432	72	214
1580	414.7324	551.0952	395	295	63	126
1581	383.8430	591.7080	302	346	65	217
1582	331.4373	649.5994	307	285	57	312
1583	508.4033	615.0740	332	290	75	175
1584	422.0286	630.4824	340	377	92	190
1585	656.0771	643.7908	378	366	94	225
1586	764.4751	729.2366	408	457	151	215
1587	484.3003	862.9658	395	440	19	256
1588	277.7458	555.1033	255	457	108	240
1589	896.8049	954.6658	766	449	85	185
1590	423.5044	731.9951	336	446	91	158
1591	542.7461	805.2981	336	444	87	239
1592	393.5098	492.4287	226	458	77	162
1593	na	na	na	0	16	na
1594	748.7224	495.6328	294	531	na	183
1595	738.9053	512.9202	303	586	24	300
1596	519.4365	595.8865	324	559	205	340
1597	505.6377	824.5242	295	565	313	286
1598	364.8433	655.3491	151	591	189	214
Min	85.3762	95.2874	18.0251	0.2000	1.2000	7.9746
Max	896.8049	954.6658	868.9788	590.7649	313.0967	339.7329
Avg	468.0035	501.1649	248.6954	246.6053	69.3842	187.1426
St Dev	174.2839	196.0164	171.4744	196.5962	57.0222	68.4043

Table 1. *(continued)*

Year	Total Credits	Total Debits	Total Income	Worsted Hall Credits	Worsted Hall Debits	Worsted Hall Income
1552	0	0.0000	0	na	na	na
1553	5470	3664.8723	1805	na	na	na
1554	2626	3826.4038	-1201	na	na	na
1555	3581	3714.3142	-133	na	na	na
1556	3098	5072.5898	-1975	na	na	na
1557	3498	2412.6362	1086	na	na	na
1558	1323	937.2432	386	na	na	na
1559	1189	0.0000	1189	na	na	na
1560	0	0.0000	0	na	na	na
1561	757	289.9478	467	na	na	na
1562	2089	2222.0549	-133	na	na	na
1563	1907	1895.9753	11	na	na	na
1564	1698	3420.3616	-1722	na	na	na
1565	3459	1609.2063	1849	na	na	na
1566	1962	2117.5979	-156	na	na	na
1567	2292	1832.9243	459	na	na	na
1568	1738	2249.1262	-511	na	na	na
1569	2267	2010.3069	256	na	na	na
1570	2468	1751.2131	717	na	na	na
1571	2397	1672.0469	724	na	na	na
1572	1236	1933.8223	-698	na	na	na
1573	2660	2597.1089	63	na	na	na
1574	1719	2449.4114	-731	na	na	na
1575	2630	2610.3772	19	na	na	na
1576	3173	2253.7668	919	25	na	25
1577	3517	3060.5312	457	50	18	32
1578	3696	3047.2969	648	44	20	23
1579	3229	3189.2153	40	75	15	59
1580	3199	2851.4893	347	9	123	-114
1581	3612	3198.7942	413	71	0	71
1582	3360	3435.8284	-75	77	na	77
1583	3692	3719.4795	-28	197	0	197
1584	3305	3184.1338	121	113	0	112
1585	3961	4571.7812	-611	184	0	184
1586	3742	4115.7383	-374	178	1	171
1587	3549	3661.9697	-113	159	20	139
1588	3219	3319.6128	-101	150	na	150
1589	3726	4850.3672	-1124	137	na	137
1590	3155	3259.7153	-104	79	8	71
1591	3745	3803.5747	-59	180	na	180
1592	2938	3168.8416	-231	81	6	74
1593	214	187.3123	27	na	na	na
1594	3707	3021.0728	686	126	na	126
1595	3426	3684.3062	-258	56	20	35
1596	4161	4564.8086	-403	53	20	33
1597	3578	5296.6172	-1718	43	20	22
1598	3365	3280.5408	84	43	20	22
Min	0.0000	0.0000	-1974.8291	8.7427	0.2000	-114.2303
Max	5469.7187	5296.6172	1849.4770	197.3813	122.9730	197.1813
Avg	2751.6954	2745.0284	6.6670	96.7394	18.4337	83.0604
St Dev	1143.8609	1308.8924	770.7614	56.4681	28.3376	72.3762

Table 1. *(continued)*

Year	Candles	Wheat & Bread	Total Debits	Miscellaneous
1552	na	na	0	0
1553	3	109	3665	2556
1554	na	137	3826	1655
1555	11	497	3714	1552
1556	7	212	5073	2882
1557	na	115	2413	1981
1558	na	na	937	87
1559	na	na	0	0
1560	na	na	0	0
1561	na	na	290	40
1562	na	na	2222	1039
1563	na	na	1896	512
1564	na	na	3420	2110
1565	7	na	1609	414
1566	7	na	2118	640
1567	13	na	1833	543
1568	na	na	2249	819
1569	na	na	2010	555
1570	5	na	1751	415
1571	16	na	1672	322
1572	4	na	1934	553
1573	13	na	2597	690
1574	1	na	2449	599
1575	10	na	2610	581
1576	10	na	2254	617
1577	10	73	3061	944
1578	10	96	3047	838
1579	10	276	3189	1095
1580	14	117	2851	804
1581	14	122	3199	1018
1582	19	149	3436	1329
1583	5	185	3719	1261
1584	10	122	3184	1020
1585	15	142	4572	1975
1586	10	538	4116	873
1587	13	353	3662	919
1588	13	268	3320	1230
1589	14	190	4850	1333
1590	16	296	3260	851
1591	14	314	3804	1094
1592	16	157	3169	1249
1593	na	36	187	135
1594	7	196	3021	762
1595	16	340	3684	970
1596	17	392	4565	1762
1597	18	514	5297	2093
1598	19	315	3281	995
Min	1.2000	35.8624		0.0000
Max	19.4625	537.9495		2881.6597
Avg	11.4269	231.8269		972.6189
St Dev	4.6899	136.0399		658.9766

Revenues (Graph 1)

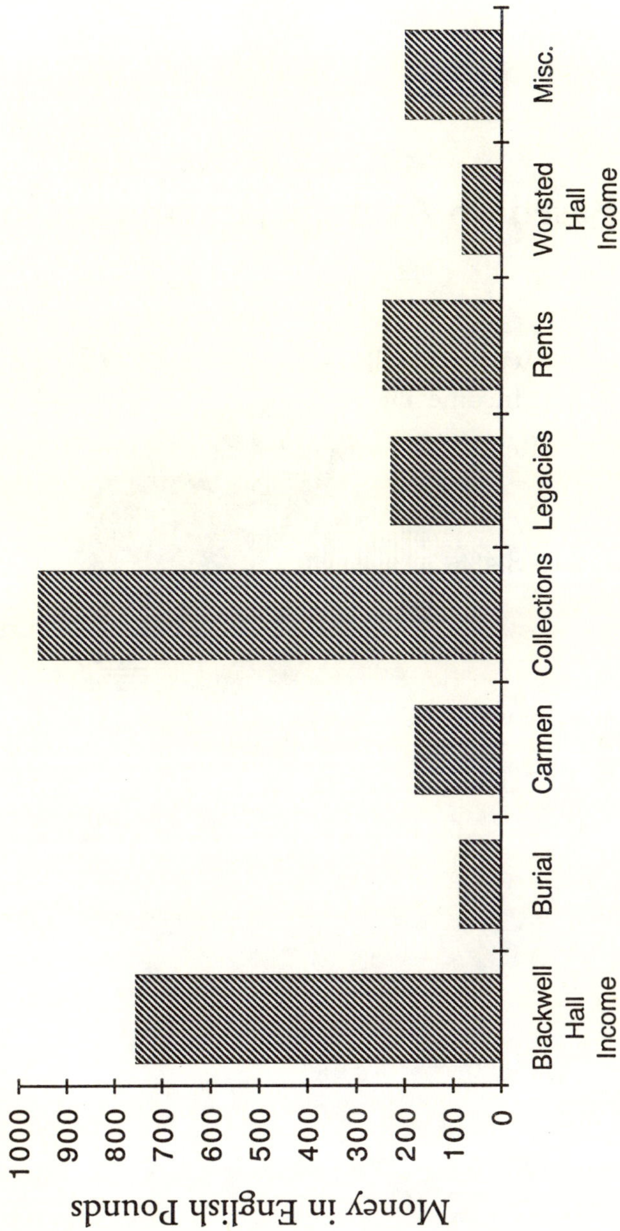

Sources of Revenue
Based on Average Revenues (Graph 2)

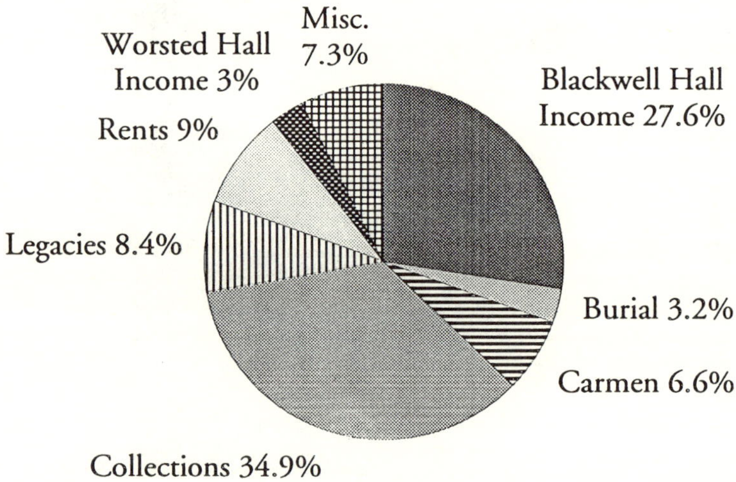

Total Credits and Debits
(Graph 3)

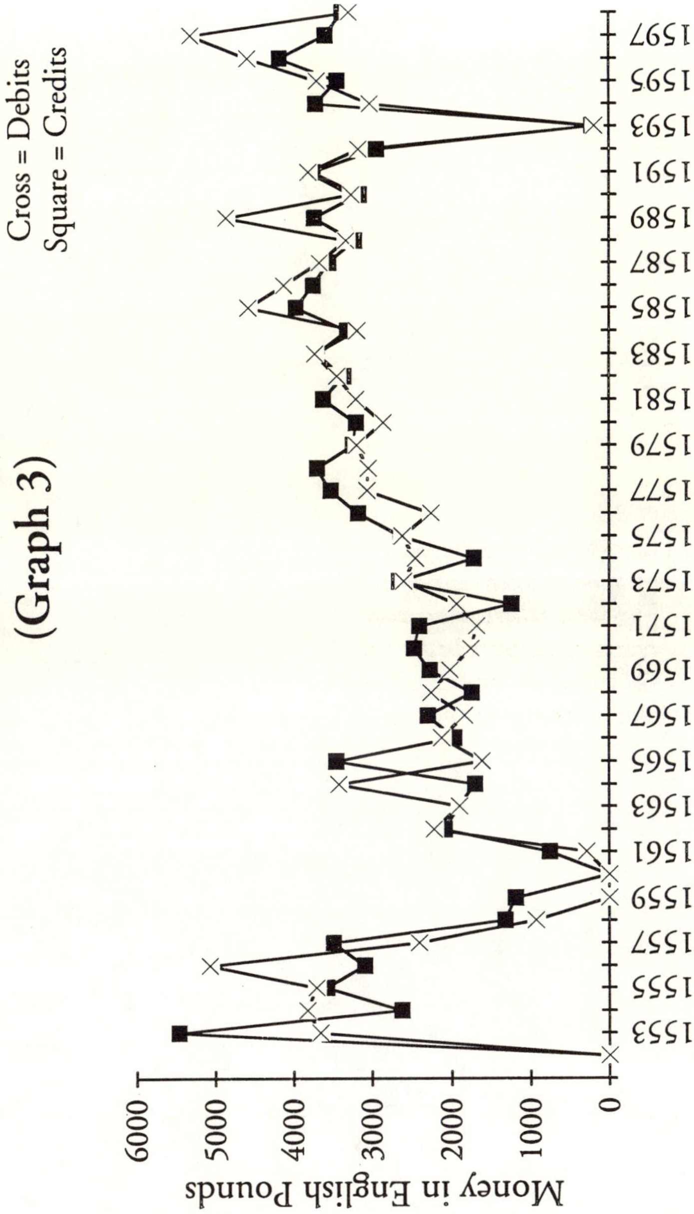

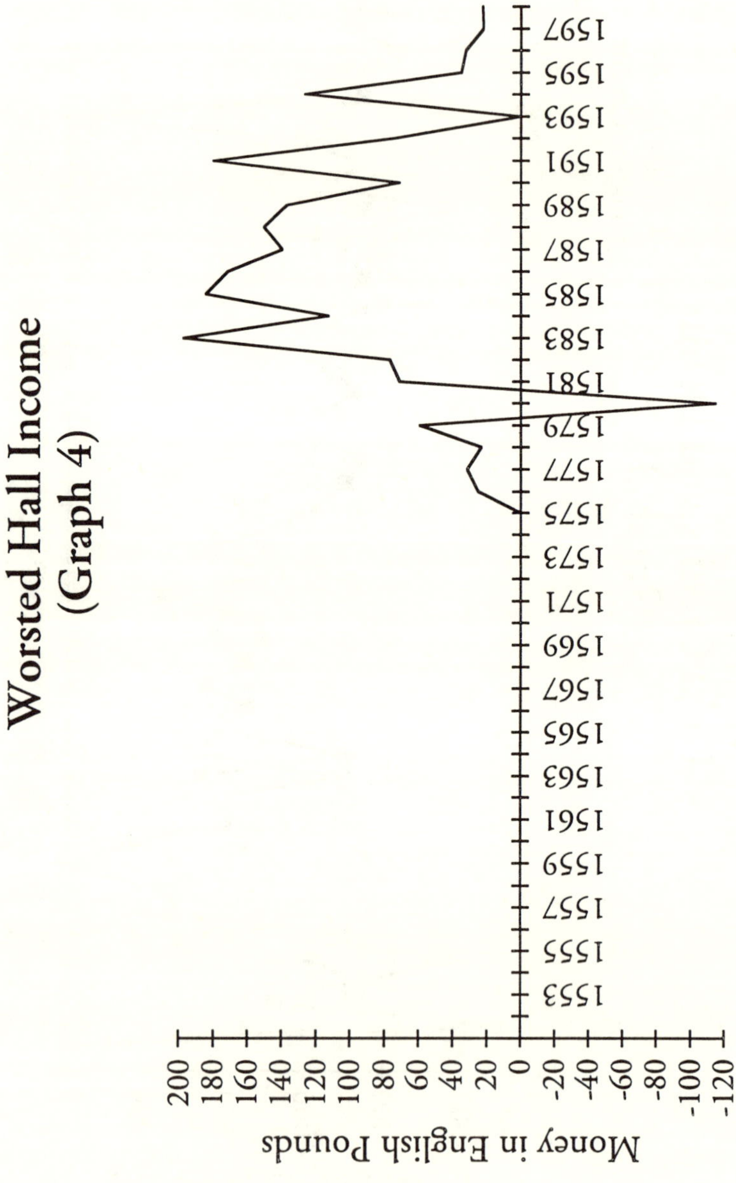
Worsted Hall Income
(Graph 4)
Money in English Pounds
200
180
160
140
120
100
80
60
40
20
0
-20
-40
-60
-80
-100
-120
1553
1555
1557
1559
1561
1563
1565
1567
1569
1571
1573
1575
1577
1579
1581
1583
1585
1587
1589
1591
1593
1595
1597

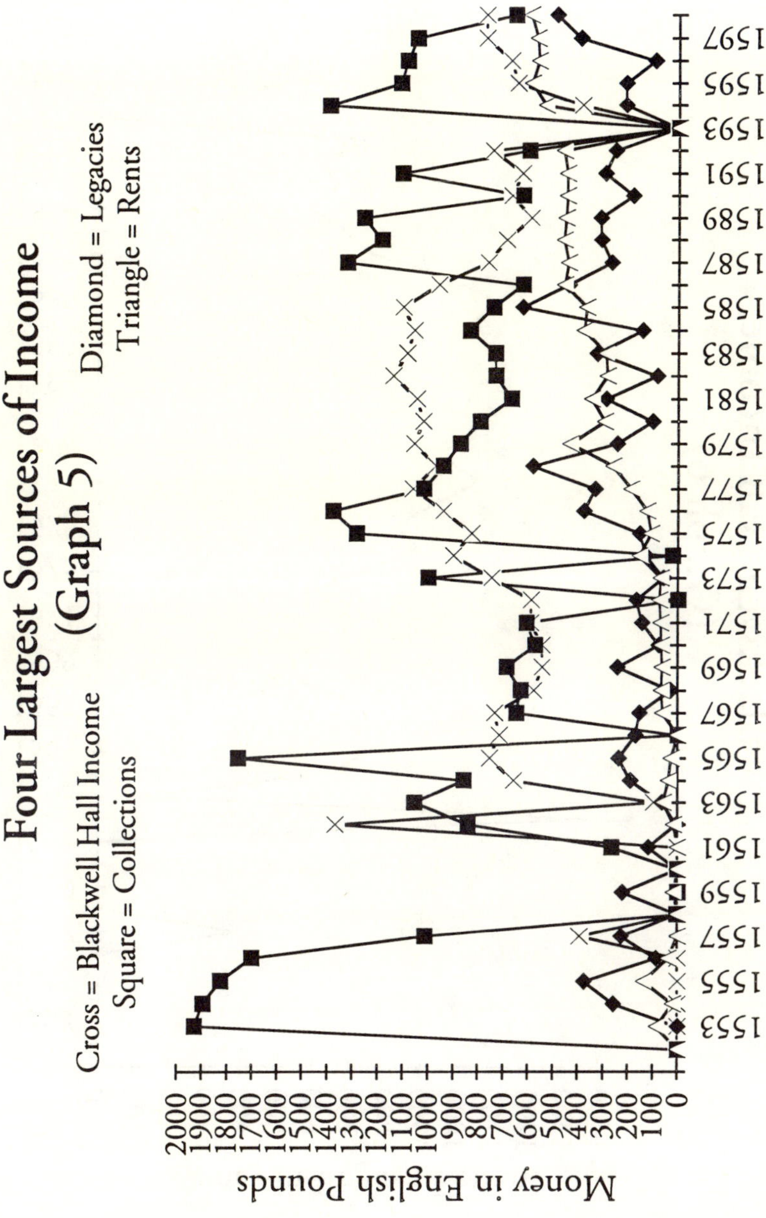
Four Largest Sources of Income
(Graph 5)
Cross = Blackwell Hall Income
Square = Collections
Diamond = Legacies
Triangle = Rents
Money in English Pounds
2000
1900
1800
1700
1600
1500
1400
1300
1200
1100
1000
900
800
700
600
500
400
300
200
100
0
1553
1555
1557
1559
1561
1563
1565
1567
1569
1571
1573
1575
1577
1579
1581
1583
1585
1587
1589
1591
1593
1595
1597

Blackwell Hall Income
(Graph 6)

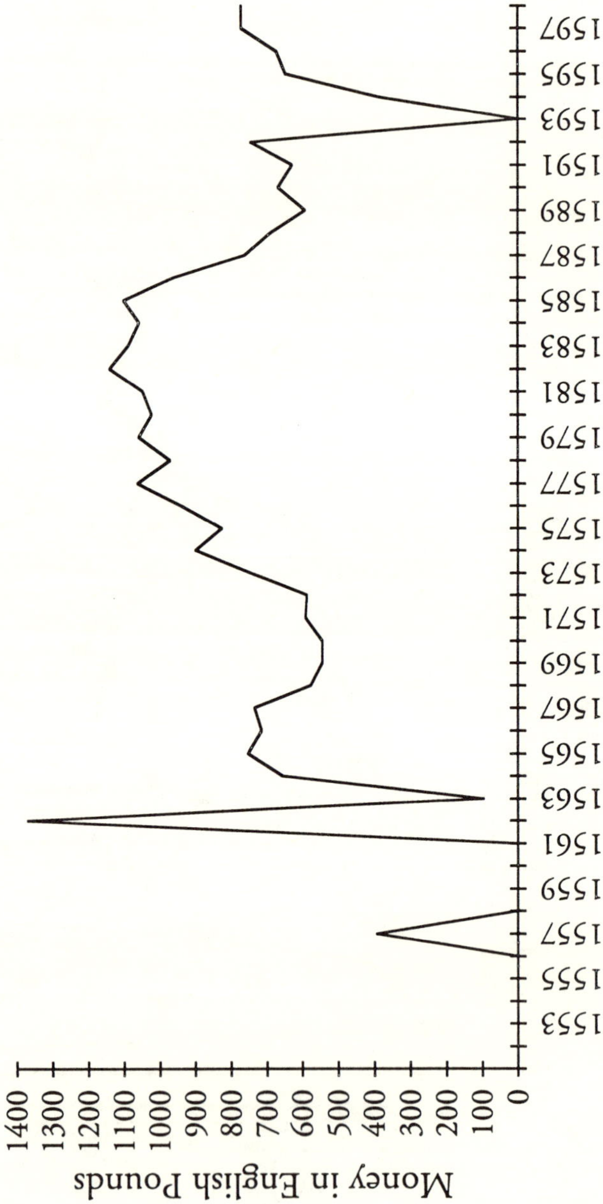

3

Revenues and Sources of Income

> A register containing all the lands, leases, and annuities that hath been given and purchased to and by Christ's Hospital in London, by good and virtuous benefactors toward ye relief of ye poor children that have been, are, and shall be by God's great goodness harbored in the same hospital. . . . But now with regard and diligence, truly gathered, and made perfect in ye time of Master Robert Cogan, now treasurer, of ye aforesaid hospital, who together with all the Governors of ye said hospital, do give God most hearty thanks, for moving the hears and minds of well disposed benefactors.
>
> —G.L., MS 12805, 1594

> that there shall be a new seal devised by the advise of Master Alderman Bowes . . . and that the same shall be always remain and be kept in this hall in the chest wherein the common seal of the City is kept and that all leases, grants, or conveyances hereafter to be made of any of the lands, tents, rents or possessions of any of the said hospitals shall always from henceforth be subscribed with the hands of the four of the governors of any of the said hospitals. . . .
>
> —G.L., MS 12806/2, 31 January 1591/92

Despite its royal foundation, Christ's Hospital did not have a sound financial foundation; the hospital's income was highly erratic. Two graphs depicting total credits and debits are especially revealing. Whereas the total annual credits of Christ's Hospital averaged £2751 13s. 11d., the total annual debits averaged £2745 7d. (see graph 3). Annual income averaged slightly more than annual expenditures: £6 13s. 4d. more was accumulated per year than spent (see table 1). The cost of the hospital's daily operations consumed almost all of its income.

The institution lingered on the edge of insolvency throughout the first five decades of its existence. The governors had great difficulty planning long-term investment strategies to improve the financial status of the hospital because there was no surfeit of funds. At the end of the fiscal year, excess monies were credited back into the general treasury to cover future expenditures. Because the governors anticipated shortfalls almost every year, investments were not given a high priority.

The volatility of the hospital's income is demonstrated by graph 5. The four largest sources of income fluctuated wildly from year to year. Patterns are difficult to discern in the data. The rise and fall of rents, legacies, collections, and Blackwell Hall's income do not correspond with one another, nor correlate with external events. For example, collections and legacies were up in 1571, but income from rents remained level and Blackwell's income fell. Of the four largest sources of income, only the income generated from rents shows a steady increase. However, rents never generated enough income to place the orphanage above constant worry about its next year's budget.

Although a few new sources of income became available, Christ's was unable to expand its revenue base with any consistency. Of new sources like Bay Hall, Blackwell Hall, burial money, carmen, and Worsted Hall, only Blackwell Hall produced a significant sum of money. Occasionally, large gifts were bestowed to Christ's Hospital, as when £500 was donated by Mistress Alice Middleton. The governors decided to invest in "some convenient purchase to be bought for this use. . . ."[1] Generous patrons were rare, however. The institution's financial condition was fragile during all the years covered by this book.

Operations at Christ's Hospital were complex and the records were meticulous. Nearly every item of income or expenditure was recorded, no matter how small the amount. The detail of these records provides a unique glimpse into the workings of a Tudor institution. The primary sources on the financial structure of Christ's Hospital are its own records as kept in the Treasurer's Account Books, two volumes covering the years 1552 to 1598.

The treasurer's accounts are divided into "charges," or credits, and "discharges," or debits. The books of Christ's were set up and kept in the same manner as the financial records of the guilds and therefore did not depart from the standard accounting practices of the time. However, the annual charges and discharges do not always coincide with the actual income or expenditures of the hospital. Account adjustments, loan or rental extensions, and unpaid debts complicate the income/expenditure structure. Accounts were compiled on an annual basis. The start of the fiscal and administrative year sometimes varied. In 1573, during his early tenure as treasurer, Hall had introduced some consistency into the practice, dating each fiscal year from Michaelmas to Michaelmas. Although the treasurer was responsible for keeping the hospital accounts, between two and four governors were appointed at the annual election each year to serve as auditors. When the treasurer totaled all charges and debts at the end of each fiscal year, the accounts were examined by the auditors. They signed their names stating what differences, if any, they found.[2]

However, as painstaking as the treasurer's accounts were, certain problems are manifest. Most distressingly, the records for the years 1552, 1558, 1560, 1561, and 1593 are incomplete. The second problem is that the entries become less specific as time goes by. For example, the method of entering transactions changed. After 1556-57, legacies were no longer recorded on specific dates, but were instead listed in a block for the entire year. Only names and amounts were recorded. A legacy for 1554–55 records the £6 13s. 4d. donated but also provides the following information: "Received by the hands of Master Hartop as the legacy of Nicholas Bull goldsmith the 19th of August 1554. . . ."[3] A more streamlined but less informative entry in 1564–65 simply records the £33 6s. 8d. "for the legacy of Sir John Lyon Knight."[4]

A third problem complicating analysis is that for five years St. Thomas Hospital's accounts were merged with Christ's Hospital. The Savoy, a former leper hospital, was given to St. Thomas Hospital under the condition that the pensions for the remaining lepers be paid by the hospital monthly, which was done from September 1552 until September 1557. Therefore, Christ's Hospital collected rents from property associated with the Savoy, and paid not only pensions to lepers but the fees to the keepers for its first five years.

The accounts at Christ's Hospital were set up so that income equaled the cash money that was counted and recorded. As a charity institution, it might be expected that gifts of bread or clothes would be common, as even modern charities receive things or services instead of cash.[5] Surprisingly, these kinds of contributions were lacking. Cash was usually given, and sometimes the donor would attach specific instructions. For example, in 1552 the hospital's accounts recorded the following: "Received of Master Blondell by the gift of diverse persons toward the making of the children pies at Christmas – 28s. 4d."[6] Money for pies was donated instead of the pies themselves or their ingredients. Some of the gifts in kind were recorded as cash values: "Received the 23rd of November 1555 of the Company of Mercers toward the apparelling of the children forty pieces of watchet containing 683 yards which amounts to the sum 66Li 13s. 3d."[7]

Gifts in kind may not have been recorded in the Account Books because they were not money and therefore not "account-able." This explains why there seems to be so few of them. However, there are two problems with this explanation. First, a few such entries do appear in the Account Books. It seems unlikely the accounts were inconsistent in recording these or any other kinds of gifts. In the fiscal year of 1582–83, the accounts listed a gift of "5 inks awarded to Christ's Hospital. . . ." The treasurer assigned no cash value to this gift, a highly unusual practice.[8] Donated items were normally assigned a cash value and faithfully entered into account.

Second, the records of the financial affairs of Christ's are painstakingly gathered with every item accounted for in detail, and presumably large numbers of gifts would not be ignored, since supplies or equipment would relieve the hospital of having to pay cash for essential articles.

Christ's Hospital received its income from a variety of sources with, of course, various impacts upon the financial health of the institution. The main sources, tabulated from the mean value of each category given to Christ's from 1552 to 1598 were, in descending order: parish collections, Blackwell Hall receipts, rents, legacies, carmen receipts, burial money, Worsted Hall receipts, Bay Hall receipts, benevolences, boxes, and annuities (see graphs 1 and 2).

Ordinary Collections was the money collected from the parishes of the City of London and comprised the largest source of income for the hospital. The smallest sum of money collected from the parishes was in 1557–58 and totaled a mere £4 11s. 4d. The largest sum of money was £1929 8s. 11d. and it is hardly surprising that this sum was amassed in 1553, the second year of the orphanage's existence, when the initial enthusiasm for Christ's was at its peak (see table 1). The average annual payment from the parishes came to £958 16s. 4d., accounting for 34.9 percent or slightly more than one-third of the total revenue (see graphs 1 and 2). Income from this source fell usually between six hundred and eleven hundred pounds. Since the parishes differed from each other in terms of wealth and available resources, any contribution made from the parishes would vary not only from parish to parish but from year to year. The unpredictability of the parish collection underscores the delicate condition of Christ's finances.

The second volume of the Minutes of the Court of Governors provides the only glimpse into gathering of income from this source and unfortunately only for the year 1562. It indicates, for example, that the collectors of St. Clement's parish located in Candlewick Ward gathered 40s. for two month's collection on "Monday the last of November"; gathered £3 for "3 month's collection" on 19 December 1562; on 21 December of the same year gathered 14s. for two month's collection; and on 17 January 1563 they gathered 40s. for two month's collection.[9] This parish, which contributed about £12 for that year, is classified as a well-to-do church by Roger Finlay.[10]

The violent fluctuations of the revenue from ordinary or monthly collections suggests that although support for Christ's Hospital and the other three hospitals was mandated by the City, each parish decided how much to donate. The parishes were obliged to support Christ's with money because it was the parishes who benefited from the services of this orphanage. It was certainly to the advantage of the parishes to support Christ's, thereby saving themselves the greater charges and headaches that would have ensued had they individually been forced to provide the care for their needy children. A more efficient level of care was certainly provided by the operation of a citywide orphanage. Nonetheless, sometimes it was necessary to prod individual parishes into meeting that obligation. Although it was not a frequent occurrence, a particular parish neglecting its monetary support of Christ's could be denied services by the hospital in the future when it attempted to place children in the orphanage. This situation confronted the parishioners of St. Michael at Queenhithe, who had requested the admission of two children to Christ's on 18 March 1592. The Court of Governors decided to admit the children under the condition of delay until "after such time as the Collectors of the parish have cleared their accompt and paid their money. . . ."[11]

The regular parish collections were not, however, the only charge upon the churches. The parishes did not abandon their responsibility to their orphans after the children were placed within the care of Christ's. They provided additional monies for the maintenance of some children: St. Giles gave £1 "towards the apparelling of 2 children admitted from the same parish";[12] and a certain amount was "Received of Thomas Jackeson churchwarden of St. Dionis Back-church toward ye apparelling of Thomas Fisher a child admitted from ye same parish. . . ."[13] Also, some conditions were established. In 1582, for instance, a notice was sent to the wards from the Lord Mayor, ordering that no child was to be admitted from the parishes unless there was a promise "to receive such child back again from the charges of the said hospital at the age of 16 years. . . ."[14]

The money collected from Blackwell Hall provided the second-largest source of income for the hospital. The first entry concerning this hall was in 1557: "Received the 13th day of April 1557 of William Wyat grocer by the assignment of my Lord Mayor and his Brethren, out of the profits of the office of Blackwell Hall – 100 Li."[15] Blackwell Hall was also known as Bakewell Hall before 1465 and stood on the east side of Guildhall Yard; "it appears to have been used as a market place for woollen clothes. Foreigners were directed to bring their woollen cloth here for sale . . . the fees from the lettings being handed over to Christ's Hospital."[16] In fact, clothworkers and merchants were not allowed to receive "any cloth in their houses till ye same [was] first pitched at Blackwell Hall & ye hallage paid for. . . ."[17] However, Christ's Hospital had to pay the fees of the officers of Blackwell Hall and the rent of the building, in addition to other charges necessary to keep the hall in operation. To get a true picture of the gross income derived from this source for the use of Christ's, the operating money must be deducted from the total receipts from Blackwell Hall. In 1564–65, the receipt from one year totaled £607 4s. 4d. The cost of operating the hall for the same year totaled £182 13s. 11d. This left £424 10s. 5d. of actual income to be used by the hospital that year. The average credits from Blackwell Hall were £815 16s. 1/4d. (see graphs 1 and 6 and table 1). The average debits were £61 7s. 10d. The necessary sums dispensed on the operations of this hall were fairly stable until the 1590s, especially when compared with the money collected from this hall.

The largest annual net income (credits minus debits) from Blackwell Hall and given to the hospital was amassed in 1562 and totaled £1369 6s. 8d. The smallest sum of money given was in 1555 and totaled a mere 13s. 4d., which was a gift and not a share in the trade that passed through the hall, as would later be the case. The average amount of money collected yearly from Blackwell was £757 12s. 4d. and accounts for 27.6 percent of total revenues (see graphs 1 and 2). Although mostly free from violent booms and slumps, the income from Blackwell Hall did noticeably vary on an annual basis depending upon the volume of the wool trade in London. This was subject to a degree of uncertainty because the trade depended not only upon the health of the wool market in England, but also in the rest of Europe. The fickleness of this revenue-producing agent was inherent in the capriciousness of the international cloth market.

Rents generated from the property owned by Christ's Hospital were an important category of income and the only source of revenue for the hospital that was potentially expandable and could provide a firm base for solvency. Rents accounted for only 9.0 percent of the average revenue for the hospital and were the third-largest source of income (see graph 2). The average collection was £231 16s. 6d. (see graph 1). The largest sum collected from this source was £537 19s. in 1598 and the lowest sum was 4s collected in 1593, which is surely a bookkeeping anomaly (see table 1). This category shows however, steady growth through the forty-eight years covered by this book and was the only significant source of income that was not unstable. The 1590s show annual income of five hundred-plus pounds generated from rents. It would be expected that as an institution becomes more established over the course of time, the properties donated from well-wishers, usually through their wills, would accumulate, and that is what happened here.

Rents were not, however, straight income. The hospital had to maintain the structures and make repairs on the buildings they owed and used as rental property. On bills dated 16 and 22 December 1581, repairs were done upon the house of Walter Rivers for the substantial cost of £10 12s. 9d.; these repairs necessitated the services of carpenters, ironmongers and tilers.[18] This same Walter Rivers, plumber, paid an annual rent of £3 6s. 8d. for his house, not terribly high when compared with the rents received from other tenants. Therefore, the fixing of Mr. Rivers's house was not just a special concession to an important tenant but was an example of a regular expense for the upkeep of the hospital's property. Therefore, the actual income from rents is lower than the figures indicate at first glance. The net income from individual properties is impossible to calculate; however, income is located in one spot in the account books under "charges," while dispersal of funds for building and ground maintenance does not necessarily appear in the same place in the same time. In fact, it tends to be scattered all over the accounting landscape. It is very difficult to adjust the annual revenues to reflect this reality because repairs were unpredictable and not a yearly expenditure. Repairs never were a large drain upon the resources of Christ's and never approached the sums of money collected as rents. Such costs were, however, prone to fluctuations.

By 1598, Christ's Hospital gathered rent from twenty-seven different endowments. It collected rents from a variety of property holdings including houses, tenements, gardens, orchards, land, messuages (houses with land attached), a tavern, and even a windmill. No two houses generated the same amount of rent. In fact, most individuals paid only a few pounds annually for their rental property. Three pounds was paid in rent by "Richard Bird for a house a year due as before. . . ."[19] Two pounds was paid in rent by "John Mules for his house and backside...."[20] Five pounds was the annual rent paid by "Master Bunnye for a tenement. . . ."[21] Only £1 rental was extracted from "Goodwife Swaine for a garden yearly. . . ."[22] The large sum of £20 was received from "master Cossen for certain lands and tenements at Horsey Down. . . ."[23] A mere 4s was the cost of renting "The great messuage or tenement called the Cock in the Hoop in the parish of St. Michael le Querne. . . ."[24] From the generosity of Richard Castler's, Samuel Haslewood rented an orchard and "backside" for £4 per annum.[25] The hospital received £10 in rent per annum from a tenant named Edmund Redding for a water mill and ground called Osier Hoop, which had been donated to the orphanage by Roger Knott.[26] The "Red Bull in Southwark," which was a tavern, was charged £12 annual rent.[27] Christ's windmill outside of "Newgate in ye parish of St. Sepulchre" brought in £5 annual rent from John Stocket.[28]

Legacies provided the fourth largest reservoir of money for the hospital. A legacy is defined simply as "A sum of money, etc. bequeathed to another: Bequest."[29] Legacies were gifts and mostly consisted of small sums of money given by individuals—usually a few shillings and not more than a few pounds. For example, 3s. 4d. was "Received the 18th day of May anno 1555 as the gift and legacy of Anthony Calverley toward the relief and help of the poor."[30] The smallest sum of money collected as a legacy was in 1562 when a mere £6 14s. was received, and the largest sum collected was in 1585 and totaled £624 11s. 11d. (see table 1). The mean annual value of legacies was £230 9s. 2d. and comprised 8.4 percent of total revenues (see graphs 1 and 2). This category of support for the hospital has the dubious distinction of being the most volatile.

Legacies that totaled ten pounds or more were separately listed in a special account called the Book of Legacies and Benefactors. The only exception in this time period to the ten pound rule was in 1561, when Sir Walter Mildmay gave yearly two pounds and twelve shillings and was still listed the Book of Legacies. Particularly revealing is the number of important donations made by women. Out of a total of 341 contributions, 47 were made by women, which is 13.8 percent of total contributions of large legacies. This percentage correlates with W. K. Jordan's conclusion that women in London from 1480 to 1660 comprised 14.88 percent of all London charitable donors.[31] Among the group of aristocratic women donors was the Lady Marquise of Winchester, who gave ten pounds to the hospital in 1586.[32] The ladies Garrett, Laxston, Raskern, Lyon, Champion, Martin, Leigh, Denney, White, and Gresham gave a total of £306 13s. 4d. from 1554 to 1583.[33] Sixteen widows are listed as having given £870 to Christ's from 1554 to 1598. In 1560, Mrs. Agnes Runt, widow, gave £100, a generous gift, which may have been an execution of her deceased husband's wishes.

(Thomas Runt, a skinner, had given £100 to Christ's in 1559, a very generous gift considering that he had no apparent connection to the hospital.) This demonstrates that women not only had enough wealth to be listed as special patrons of the hospital but that they were not reluctant about supporting causes they believed to be worthwhile.

Most of the male benefactors listed in the Book of Legacies fall into three categories: governors of the hospitals, aldermen and city officials, and guild members. In 1598, Richard Venables, merchant tailor, gave Christ's the sum of £40 even though he seems to have been more closely connected to St. Bartholomew's Hospital, where he served as a governor in 1592–93 and 1595–96.[34] Another generous donor was Peter Haughton, who gave £150 in 1597 when he served as an alderman; he had formerly been a sheriff in 1593.[35] The most interesting entry in the Book of Legacies describes Robert Marriott, who donated £10 in 1591, as "Clerk and sometimes a child of this house." When he was seventeen, Robert Marriott was discharged from the hospital (on 17 September 1563) to the care of his parents.[36] It is indicative of the quality of care given to the children that one of its former charges not only seems to have prospered enough but also to have retained enough fondness for his former home to make a sizable gift. However, most of the legacies were small gifts, as evidenced by the "Legacies Adjusted" column in table 1.

The money generated from the carmen account was the fifth-largest source of income for the hospital. The carmen's money provided an average of £180 10s. This is especially impressive when it is considered that the carmen account only became a source of revenue in 1582/83. The smallest amount of money collected was £112 12s. 10d. in 1588 and the largest amount of money collected was £275 3s. 6d. in 1594 (see table 1). The carmen account encompasses 6.6 percent of total income for Christ's and provided fairly reliable funding (see graph 2).

> In 1582 the City provided another source of income, when the Court of Aldermen decreed "that the Treasurer and Governors of Christ's Hospital shall from henceforth have the rule, charge, oversight, and government of all the Carts, Cars and Carmen . . .all which benefit commodity and profits rising or coming by the same to be employed only to the relief of the poor children within the same Hospital."[37]

The carmen, employed in "Her Majesty's service" with their horses and carts, were crucial to the smooth running of the economy of Tudor London.[38] Goods did not move in, out, or around the City without the carmen.

> The carmen undertook to keep the streets clean and to carry goods at rates fixed by the city. . . . At the end of the century the number of licensed cars was fixed at 400. . . .The right to one of these 400 strands or car-rooms, as they were called, came to be regarded as the chattel of the holder...The city, however, was unwilling to admit this complete freehold of the carmen, and placed them in a kind of feudal relation to the Governor of Christ's Hospital, who became entitled to a yearly rent for each licence and a fine when it was transferred.[39]

Christ's was responsible for regulation of the affairs of the carmen, which was a condition for the City assigning money from this source of funding to the hospital. In order to maintain appropriate supervision, Christ's kept the Annual Car Accounts for the purpose of

> containing the accompts of all such profits and sums of money as do arise and grow every year yearly to Christ's Hospital in London of all the Car rooms that are in tenure as well of the woodmongers, as of all the Carmen, freemen, & foreigners within the City of London and liberties thereof. . . .[40]

This revenue-producing account provided a steady and reliable flow of income.

Burial money started producing income for Christ's in 1570–71 and so was a latecomer to the economic fabric of the hospital. It was the sixth-largest source of income, but was not a large moneymaker; most of the collected sums varied between £50 and £130. The only year that burial money contributed more than £150 was in 1596–97, and this contribution amounted to £193 16s. 4d. The smallest sum of burial money collected was £13 in 1571 (see table 1). Money bestowed upon the hospital from this source averaged £86 12s. 10d. and accounted for 3.2 percent of its total revenue (see graphs 1 and 2). This money was generated from the children acting as mourners and singing at the funerals of London citizens. "To parade one's beneficiaries at one's own funeral was an expression of pride, even if the spectacle could only be enjoyed in the imagination of the deceased before he died."[41] Burial money, given usually in amounts of £1 or £2, was donated to the hospital "for the burial of Master Hollenshead a vintner."[42] In the same year £1 was donated "for the burial of Mistress Greene a poulter's wife" and the same figure was also given "for the burial of Master Hide one of ye Lord Mayor officers."[43] The only condition placed upon the participation of the children seems to be that the gift was a cash donation. The Court of Aldermen stated "that it shall be lawful for the treasurer and governors of Christ's Hospital to permit and suffer all such children of the same hospital as are new out of the same either in the city or in the country to go to the burial of such persons as shall give anything to the maintenance of the same hospital."[44] The most interesting funeral that Christ's children attended was that of Lord Mayor Skinner, who had died while in office and who had served as a governor of the hospital since 1588. "The Children of the hospital" were a conspicuous part of the procession after Master Marshall Reade and his men and before conductors Allen and Boone.[45] As a source of income, burial money was highly unstable because it relied upon a certain number of well-to-do citizens dying each year, who would also make donations to the hospital.

Worsted Hall was a custom hall, similar to Blackwell Hall, through which cloth was exchanged within London. It can be presumed that Worsted Hall got its name from trading in worsted wool, which was the most common cloth for making stockings. Worsted cloth is defined as "A closely twisted yarn made of long-staple wool in which the fibres are arranged to lie parallel to each other. Later, a fine and soft woollen yarn used for knitting and embroidery."[46] Worsted Hall provided the seventh-largest concentration of money given to Christ's Hospital and accounted for 3.0 percent of its income (see graph 2). This hall started as an income source in 1576.

Like Blackwell Hall, Worsted Hall had a special relationship with Christ's; the expenses of running the hall were borne by the hospital. Why this custom hall came under the jurisdiction of an orphanage is never explained in the records. One could speculate that the corporation may have felt that putting Blackwell, Worsted, and Bay Halls under the supervision of Christ's had a twofold advantage to the City. First, the fines and taxes from these halls were a painless way to support the hospital. Secondly, the governors of Christ's Hospital would oversee hall operations and would thereby relieve the overburdened Court of Aldermen of the headache of managing yet another city institution. The largest collection from Worsted came to £197 3s. 7d. in 1583. The average income from this hall was £83 1s. 1d. The smallest sum was a minus £114 4s. 8d. in 1580 (see table 1). In that year, the income from Worsted was only £8 14s. 10d. and the expenses were considerably larger at £122 19s. 6d. The expenses or debits had to be deducted from the income or credits (see graph 4 and table 1). This illustrates the possibility that by paying the operational expenses for Blackwell and Worsted Halls, the potential of losing money from a revenue source was a present danger for Christ's. However, apart from the above-mentioned case, the expenses involved in running Worsted Hall were minimal and fairly constant, never rising above the £30 mark. The money from Worsted Hall, as is the case with Blackwell Hall, was unpredictable because it relied upon the quantity of wool brought into London for sale, which was not constant. In 1590 approximately £80 was garnered from this source, while the following year produced almost double that amount.

Bay Hall was yet another hall functioning as a depot for cloth trading within the city by "strangers." Bay Hall was the place that non-Londoners came "for hallege of Bays etc. being brought, and pitched. . . ."[47] Bays are a type of wool cloth probably named after its reddish-brown color and presumably most of the wool that passed through this hall was in bays cloth.[48] Receipts from Bay Hall started flowing into Christ's in the fiscal year of 1575–76. The mean value of income is £73 15s. 5d., constituting the eighth-largest source of income. The smallest sum of money collected from this hall was £9 5s. 10d. in 1594. The largest sum gathered was £186 1s. 3d. in 1580 (see table 1). The income generated from this area forms part of a miscellaneous category on graphs 1 and 2. Together with benevolence, annuities, and boxes, it generated 7.3 percent of total income (see graph 2).[49] Bay Hall's contribution to Christ's revenue was unreliable.

The benevolence category was a grab bag of widely assorted donations that defy quick or easy characterization. It was basically a compilation of gifts or contributions that were not really appropriately placed under another heading. Benevolence constitutes the most diverse category of income for the hospital and provides some insight into the motivations of donors who made gifts to the hospital. A benevolence is simply described as "an act of kindness; a gift of money, a charitable contribution."[50] Benevolences provided an average income of £71 9s. 9d. The largest sum of money given to Christ's was in 1555 and amounted to £540 4s. 2d. The smallest sum of money recorded from this source was £14 7s. 8d. in 1584 (see table 1). Together with annuities, boxes, and Bay Hall, benevolences accounted for only 7.3 percent of income (see graph 2). It was a stable source of funding, only rising above £100 upon seven occasions and mostly hovering between the £40 and £50 mark.

Some of the benevolence items were simply gifts made to the orphanage by a group. Five pounds was given "of the gift of the Lords of the Parliament";[51] £2 "of the inhabitants in the BlackFriars";[52] and £13 "Received of the merchants of the Stylliard."[53]

Benevolence income, however, was usually bestowed by individuals. Two shillings were donated "of the gift of the Lady Gresham's Maid."[54]

Two pounds was "of the gift of a party unknown."[55] One pound from "the Lady Marquise of Winchester" also was given as a benevolence.[56] Some benevolences were given on a somewhat regular basis but not always for the same sum of money. Such were the gifts "of Master Nowell Dean of Paul's" for £3 6s. 8d. and the "Bishop of London" for £4.[57] In the previous year, the bishop of London had only donated £1.[58]

Benevolences were given to Christ's as an offering of thanksgiving upon the safe return from a hazardous journey. One pound five shillings was received "Of the gift of certain mariners that went afishing to the New Found Land."[59] Even more grateful was a Master Gureney, who presented to the hospital £5: "his goods assumed being in the peril on the sea and could not have the same so assured, therefore upon the safe arrival thereof . . ."[60] Sometimes benevolences were given as a prayer offering during illness: "Received of Master Heardson Alderman as his gift in the extremity of his sickness towards the relief of the poor." He gave the large sum of £40.[61]

Another common occasion for bestowing a benevolence upon Christ's Hospital was upon the admission of a child into the hospital. The following entry of the receipt of £1 "from the Lord Mayor and Court of Alderman with a man child called Thomas Dale" was an unusual act of charity on the Lord Mayor's part, for it was within his jurisdiction to order the admission of any child into the hospital with or without money, although he did not normally interfere with the daily operation of the orphanage.[62] There is no entry in the minutes of court meetings discussing Thomas Dale's admission. The only information is contained in the Children's Register, which simply records for 19 July 1572, "Thomas Dale, 8 (Court of Aldermen)."[63] This entry contains just the basic information that this child was named Thomas Dale, that he was eight years old at the time of admission, and that he was sent thither by the Court of Aldermen. It is difficult to ascertain if this child was accorded special consideration or not. An award of money might have been a condition of the admission of a particular child, but this is by no means clear. Ten shillings was "Received of Edmond Phillips grocer for part of 20s promised by him with the admission of William Phillips his brother's child. . . ."[64] London parishes were also inclined to donate a benevolence with a child. St. Albans parish gave £4 6d. when a child was admitted into the hospital.[65] It was not only the parishes or organs of city government that found money to ease a child into the orphanage. A generous sum of £5 was "Received of the King of Portugal's ambassador with a poor infant laid at his gate in Tower Street. . . ."[66]

To obtain a lease for property held by the hospital, it was often necessary to pay a fine. William Gale, barber surgeon, paid 10s "for the fine of a lease. . . ."[67] Some of the fines charged by the City were donated to Christ's as a benevolence. The chamberlain of London sent in a fine of £200 received of Robert Harding and Jeffrey Walkrdon, who elected to pay money in lieu of serving as sheriff: "for not taking upon them the office of Sheriff. . . ."[68] Various other fines also found their way into the orphanage. In 1569 £10 19s. was divided between St. Thomas, Bridewell, and Christ's as fines paid by "men that use false measures and such like."[69] Before burial money became a separate category in the 1570–71 fiscal year, these collections were recorded as benevolences. Twelve pence was "Received of Master Burfam the 7th of May 1555 as his gift to 12 children attending upon the burial of his wife. . . ."[70] Then there were those benevolences that were highly unusual. The sum of £25 was bestowed as a benevolence as a "forfeiture of goods that was made by one of [the] tenants by committing a murder within the liberty of St. Thomas Hospital's close."[71] Five shillings were given "of Master Box treasurer toward ye printing ye psalmes. . . ."[72]

Benevolences were also small amounts of income produced by the sale of various things from the hospital. A sum of £3 15s. 8d. was presented to the treasury by the matron "for old linen rags sold, & for certain bone lace. . . ."[73] Money received from parish boxes found their way into Christ's as benevolences after they were no longer figured into box money. Thus it says that 7s. 3d. came "of the Box from Portsoken for last year. . . ."[74] Whatever the specific gifts or their intended purposes, the benevolences that found their way into the treasury of Christ's Hospital seemed to be anything but simply a "gift of money or charitable contribution."

As the name suggests, box money came from boxes located throughout the city as the Tudor equivalent of a "poor box." Originally there were a mayor's box, a matron's box, Blackwell Hall's box, Merchant Adventurers' box, Communion boxes in the parishes, the wardmote inquest boxes, and the four boxes in Christ's Hospital itself. After the first few years of the hospital's existence, only the four boxes in the hospital itself and the boxes in the wardmote inquests generated sums of any significance. The most important boxes were the ones residing at the wardmote inquests in each ward; they functioned as a reservoir for fines levied by the wards.[75] For example, "The money gathered for Christ's Hospital" from Cornhill Wardmote ranged from around 32s. to 19s.[76] The mean value of money engendered from all box sources was £37 6d. The largest contribution from the various boxes was in 1555 and amounted to £84 19s. 4d. The smallest sum of money only grossed £8 1s. 3d. for the orphanage in 1552 (see table 1). Boxes, along with benevolences, annuities, and Bay Hall, comprised 7.3 percent of total income (see graph 2). Box money was never an important income-generating device but provided a reliable source of money, generally falling between £25 and £50 per annum.

Annuities are, as the name suggests, funds that are set up to be given on a year-to-year basis: "a yearly alowance or income."[77] People would donate an amount of money and in return would get a small yearly allowance. Annuities also fell within the miscellaneous category. The average sum of money collected from this source totaled £18 13s. 4d. The smallest sum of money gathered from this source was £1 4s. 4d. in 1570. The largest sum was £79 15s. 9d., collected in 1596 (see table 1). Annuities were given in small amounts, and the total greatly varied on an annual basis, furnishing the least important source of regular income.

Some income was highly irregular in nature. Such small, unexpected pecuniary resources did not fall into the eleven regular categories of income already examined. For example, the sale of iron provided 30s. in the 1561-62 fiscal year.[78] In 1597–98 the sale of old rags by the matron netted 15s. 7d., which was turned over for the use of the hospital.[79] Money was sometimes collected for unusual purposes; thus £145 3s. 2d. was collected in March and April of 1553 for the paving of the town ditch.

Given the delicate and variable nature of the hospital's income, a constant concern over money was inevitable. Christ's Hospital operated on the brink of economic collapse every year. Given the desperate straits it found itself in, the fact that the hospital didn't disappear during the bad economic times of the 1590s is surprising. The entire economy of England was in crisis in the 1590s: this decade registered the highest prices of the century for wool and wheat while wages were at their lowest point.[80] Voluntary gifts diminish in bad times, while the demand for services increases.

There were only two ways that the governors could reduce adverse balances in the institution's financial accounts. They could either reduce the number of people dependent upon the hospital or increase the revenues. In fact, these two goals were not incompatible and frequently worked together as a strategy to ease the problem. An example of an attempt to decrease the number of children served occurred on 18 December 1591, when the Court of Governors ordered that foundlings were not to be admitted. The governors observe, "[I]t is found by experience that the admitting of a few of these children hath drawn the enterprise of a number more of those practices than ever would have been attempted had not been the compassion used in accepting of such in the beginning. . . ."[81] This is a distress signal on the part of the governors, for they had long felt a Christian obligation towards such unfortunate children, who had been admitted as a matter of policy into the orphanage since its founding. It was a measure of the economic hardship of the 1590s that the hospital considered changing its established tradition of compassion towards these children. Earlier the same month, when Master Morgan, the Queen's apothecary, attempted to gain entry to Christ's for a child, the governors ordered the treasurer to write a letter "informing him of the great want of this house and how greatly it is overcharged and pray him to have patience until the state of this house be mended."[82] It is a further indication of the severe distress felt by Christ's that in 1595 the governors stated that no further petitions from the parishes for admission of children would be considered between July and "Bartholomewtide [24 August] next coming or until that shall please God things are become more cheaper."[83] This unusual decision was prompted by "ye great charges of this house. . . ."[84] Extraordinary stress is revealed by the governor's request in 1598 to the Lord Mayor not to order the admission of children "until this house shall be made more able to grant by order of Court admission. . . ."[85]

In addition to addressing the matter of children, the governors felt obliged to take any action deemed necessary to keep the poor out of the city. As will be shown, it was not only children that benefited directly from the charity of Christ's Hospital. Pensions were also given to needy and destitute adults who did not necessarily have children. So any attempt to lessen the burden upon the hospital through the reduction of the number of poor who might lay a claim to the bounty of the orphanage was undertaken to help ease its financial burden. The situation was deemed serious enough in the fall of 1590 to appoint special committees from the four hospitals "to consider of a course for the clearing of this city of London of rogues, beggars, and children vagrants."[86]

In addition, the governors started to devote a great deal of effort to identifying and locating the fathers of illegitimate children. They initiated harsh measures against fathers who abandoned their illegitimate children. This was clearly an attempt to force these men to assume their paternal responsibilities and thus relieve the city of the cost of caring for their children.

More energy was devoted to keeping their revenues from shrinking than to attempting to augment revenues from previously untapped sources or attempting to reduce spending. The minutes from the governors' court demonstrate the hysteria felt over the declining revenues from Blackwell Hall. As already noted, Blackwell Hall constituted the second-largest source of income to the hospital, and the governors looked closely into any matter that affected the flow of money from Blackwell or its operating efficiency. There seems to be good reason for the governors' concern over the condition of Blackwell Hall. Starting in 1587, the hospital's income from this source started a noticeable decline that didn't abate in the next decade. When compared with its previous performance, the decline was alarming. Starting in 1574, Blackwell Hall produced over £800 per annum for Christ's treasury. From 1577to 1585, it generated more than £1000 per annum. At the same time that revenues from this hall were increasing, the expense of maintaining it rose. The hospital administrators devoted a great deal of time and effort to locate the source of the problem, and they concluded that bad management and outright corruption by hall officials were to blame. Richard Oliver, one of the clerks of Blackwell Hall, was under constant scrutiny from the governors until his final dismissal on 3 October 1597, though he seems to have been dismissed before that and subsequently reinstated. As early as March 1595 he was warned not to meddle in the affairs of the hospital.[87] Richard Oliver, Morgan Flewellen, and Oliver Jones were called to explain the discrepancies in their accounts before the governors. But whether they were incompetent or just plain corrupt is unclear; certainly the temptation to accept payment under the table for overlooking the regular custom duties must have been great. The governors placed Blackwell Hall under closer supervision by ordering that the account books be brought in to be examined by the treasurer on every Monday.[88] Further supervision was deemed necessary, and in 1598 five governors were appointed as overseers: "And these governors according to their wisdoms to give their attendance at Blackwell Hall to ye purpose aforesaid at such times & days of market as is holden & kept in ye said Blackwell Hall."[89] Despite the efforts of the governors to bolster receipts from Blackwell Hall, they were apparently ineffectual, for in 1598 only £769 2s. 2d. was given over to Christ's Hospital. The governors were concerned with good reason; while the money received from Blackwell Hall showed a distinctive downward spiral, the expense of running Christ's had undergone a definite upward trend.

In fact, since the economic health of Blackwell Hall required the economic health of the wool trade, it is more probable that this "decay of the profits" was a result of the decay of the wool trade and the decay of the economy as a whole. The 1590s saw the highest prices for wool in the sixteenth century and high prices would have served to decrease the demand for wool, thus lessening the trade.[90]

Other measures were tried to ensure collection of money due to Christ's. Hospital officials called scruteners were appointed and instructed "diligently to search and inquire from time to time for all such gifts, legacies and bequests . . . given or bequeathed to the succor and comfort of the poor harbored in Christ's Hospital. . . ."[91] The job of the scruteners was to ensure that any money allotted to Christ's through gifts or wills was promptly collected and turned over to the treasurer. In addition, the scruteners were instructed to request that the bishop of London inspire his ministers to plead with their parishioner "to yield & give to the maintenance of the said hospital weekly. . . ."[92]

As a part of their watchful vigilance over declining revenues, the governors reproached people for not paying their share of relief to the poor. Marmeduke Franke, a shoemaker, had not paid and was "now upon the knowledge of his fault forgiven and . . . granted to the poor 2d. weekly."[93] It wasn't just individuals who were called by the governors to account for their lack of payment; churches were also faulted. "Certain parishes were appointed to be sent for before the Governors who have withdrawn their charity for the poor."[94] Presumably, just a summons to appear before the Court of Governors loosened the purses of those concerned.

At a court meeting in November of 1592, six governors were appointed to go inform the Lord Mayor and the Court of Aldermen of "The great decay of the estate of this house. . . ."[95] These representatives were instructed to inform them that the situation was so acute "and to give them to understand that Master Treasurer is ready to give up the keys."[96] A complaint was received from the country nurses in 1596 that illustrates their concern with their failing resources. They write about "ye dearth of this year & of ye long time of scarceness & their wages being not sufficiently to maintain & continue their nurseries. . . ."[97] The treasurer was directed to provide what relief he felt necessary, but not to increase the wages of the nurses. Desperation is again apparent when in 1598 the governors agreed to attempt to acquire a loan of £800 from the Lord Mayor to cover money already spent on "necessary expenses."[98] A commission from Christ's composed of seven governors and Master Cogan, the treasurer, was selected to present the petition.

Assessing the exact dimensions of the fiscal crises confronting Christ's Hospital is formidable, for the Treasurer's Accounts present a monetary nightmare. Clearly, however, the institution hovered every year on the brink of financial destitution. The governors' panic was not unjustified; as their expenditures were rising, income was falling, placing the institution in danger of extinction. From 1588 until 1598, the hospital was in the red for seven out of the ten years. The orphanage survived only because its governors refused to allow it to close its doors; somehow, the money to continue operations was always found. That Christ's was able to expand the sources of revenue, if only in a limited way, was an important indication of the commitment of the governors and the corporation. The only sound revenue enhancement strategy would have been to purchase property in the rapidly growing city, but Christ's lacked the necessary cash and generous benefactors could not be relied upon for that purpose. But then again, if Christ's Hospital had acquired large holdings of property, it might not have been much different from the English Catholic Church, whose convents and monasteries seldom went broke dispensing their alms to orphans, widows, and the poor. Maybe forcing the hospital to rely constantly upon the goodwill of the citizens of London served as a guarantee that if the institution fell into disfavor or no longer filled the need of Londoners, it would dissolve quickly and not be so wealthy that it could use its wealth as a power base. Whether it was the personal interest of its governors, their relentless dedication, their substantial wealth and influence, the overwhelming need for an institution like Christ's Hospital, or a combination of all of these, the orphanage weathered the fiscal maelstrom of the century's end and continued its operation.

The other half of the fiscal balance sheet, the expenditures, is studied next. As chapter 4 demonstrates, the hospital's disbursements are even more complicated than the picture presented here by Christ's income-generating structure.

4

Expenditures: The Cost of Running Christ's Hospital

> A good remembrance to be observed that other hospitals in London do spend ye profits of their lands upon foul persons country people and such like but very little upon citizens and Londoners which this house altogether doth relieve and comfort in ye best poor kind of people aged and infants.
>
> —Court of Governors (1599)

Given the difficulties the hospital faced with sustaining an adequate amount of revenue, the question naturally arises as to the level of care provided to the children and whether they suffered in any way when money was in short supply. Were the children of Christ's Hospital fed gruel and water and clothed in rags? As this chapter will show, the hospital's generous expenditures upon food, clothing, and other items for the children is strong evidence that the youngsters were well cared for, physically and spiritually.

The expenditures of the hospital can be roughly divided into regular, semiregular, and extraordinary expenses. For regular expenses there are entries almost every year in the account books. That does not, however, mean that those expenditures classified here as irregular were not purchased on a regular basis by the hospital. Such expenditures may have been regularly purchased but were lumped together into the ubiquitous category of "necessaries." In the Treasurer's Account Books, the earlier entries are more detailed. Therefore, those items that are classed as semiregular may be more a reflection of the manner of record-keeping than lack of routine purchase and consumption.

What role inflation played in the prices paid for the assorted items is a complex question that is beyond the scope of this study. The record of regular expenditures can shed little light on the economic conditions of Londoners in the sixteenth century. The expenditures on food and other commodities purchased increased over the period covered by this study because the number of children cared for by Christ's also increased over the same period of time.

The idiosyncrasies of the Treasurer's Account Books make it almost impossible to detail with much precision who decided what was to be spent and the procedure by which these decisions were implemented. It is difficult to gauge how much spending was at the discretion of the treasurer and how much was mandated by the governors. The Minutes of the Court of Governors suggests that the treasurer possessed some authority for purchasing the routine necessities for the hospital, while unusual discharges probably had to be approved by the body of governors. The governors exercised control over the dispersal of funds and indirectly regulated the people who received assistance from Christ's.

Christ's Hospital bought hundreds of items to clothe, feed, and otherwise tend to the needs of its charges. Such regular expenditures are here aggregated into the following eight general categories: nursing, necessaries, food, pensions, clothing, staff, fuel, and candles.

Payments to the nurses and to the staff constituted the single most important regular expenditure of Christ's Hospital.[1] The cost of nursing accounts for 25.3 percent of the regular expenditures (see graph 8). The average annual sum expended upon nursing was £501 3s. 4d.[2] The largest cost was £954 13s. 4d. in 1589 and the smallest cost was £95 5s. 9d. in 1561 (see table 1). The cost of nursing covered both in-house staff and "country nurses." The country nurses were actually wet nurses, who cared for the infants and young children outside the confines of Christ's. These children were not returned to be housed within the hospital until they reached the age of four years. Payments to wet nurses included not only their wages but also money for the needs of their charges. The in-house nursing staff received their wages under "nursing" but received additional allotments (board wages) to cover their food.

As explained in chapter 2, the matron was the head nurse and the hospital official directly in charge of, and responsible for, the children. The matron received a salary and additional benefits. The matron's salary of 10s. 8d. was "paid unto her for her own diet and for her maidens for 2 weeks. . . . "[3] Occasional needed items were paid for out of her pocket, and she was later reimbursed. For example, 11s was for such items as "medicines . . . soap ashes and diverse other things, as bowls, brooms, earthen pots. . . ."[4] In addition to wages and board wages, the matron and nurses also received a uniform. A total of £7 17s. 8d. was expended for staff liveries, no doubt as part of the Easter Spittle Sermon: "Liveries for ye matron, nurses and ye 2

Regular Expenditures #1
(Graph 7)

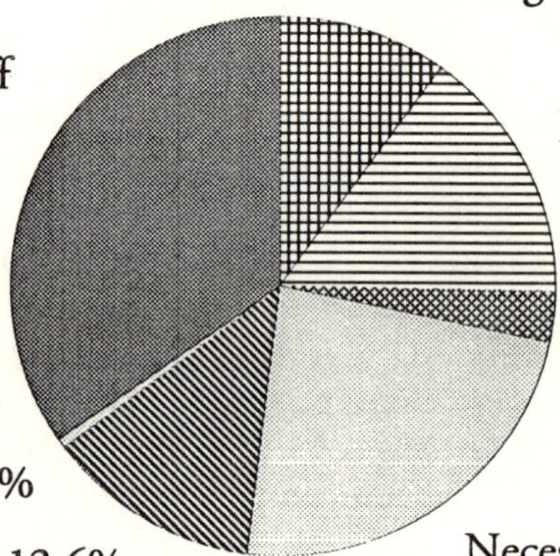

Regular Expenditures #2 (Graph 8)

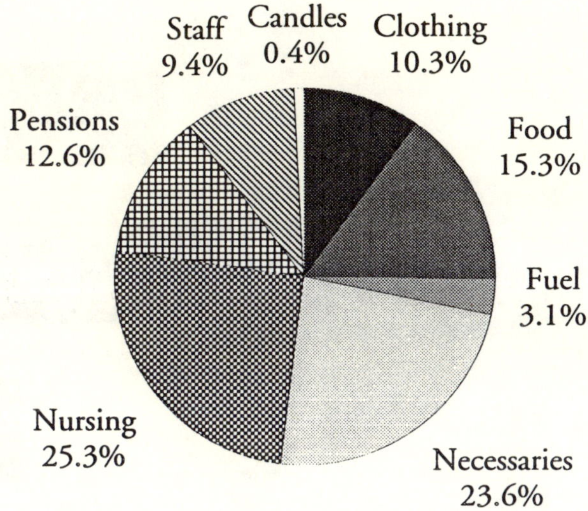

Regular Expenditures #1
(Graph 9)

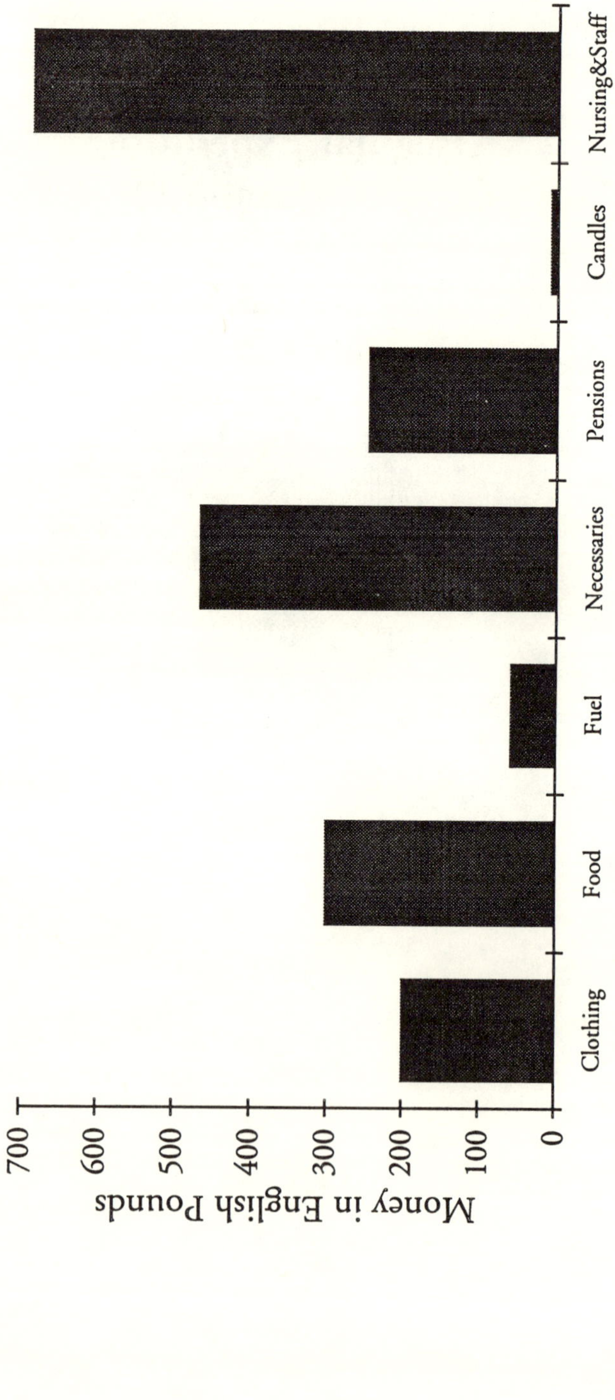

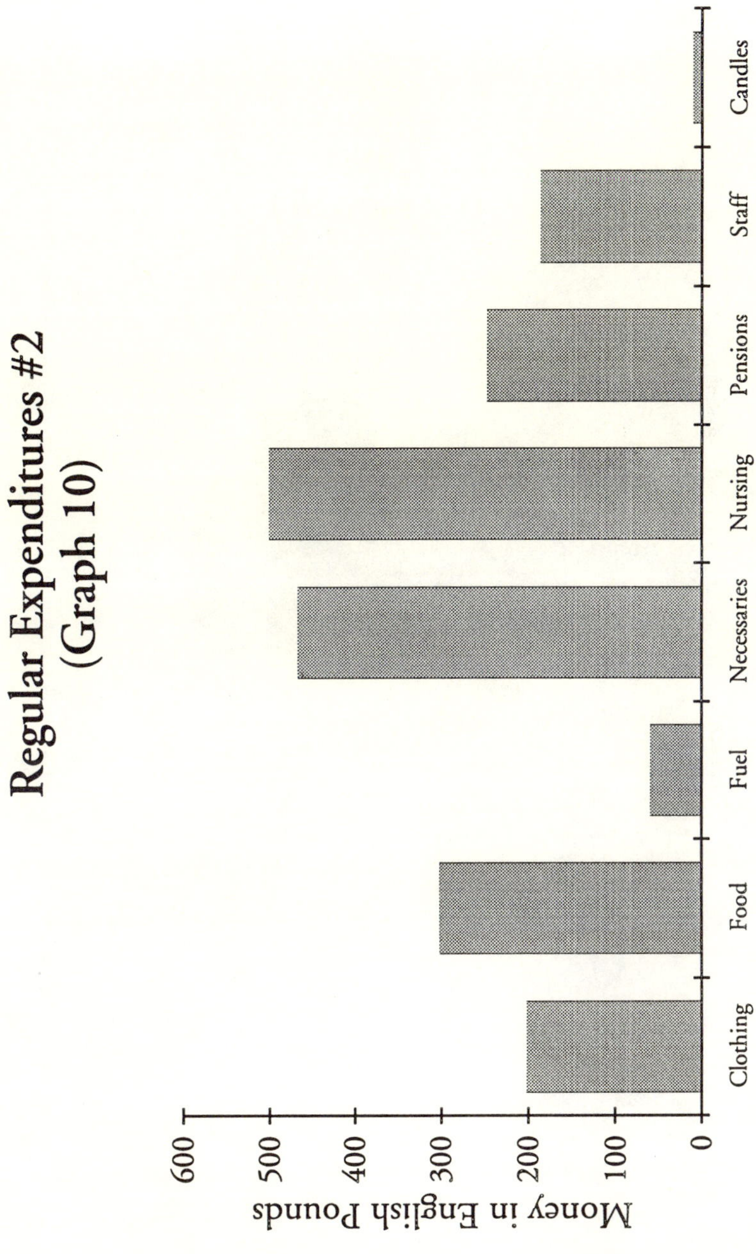
Regular Expenditures #2
(Graph 10)
Money in English Pounds
0
100
200
300
400
500
600
Clothing
Food
Fuel
Necessaries
Nursing
Pensions
Staff
Candles

Food
(Graph 11)

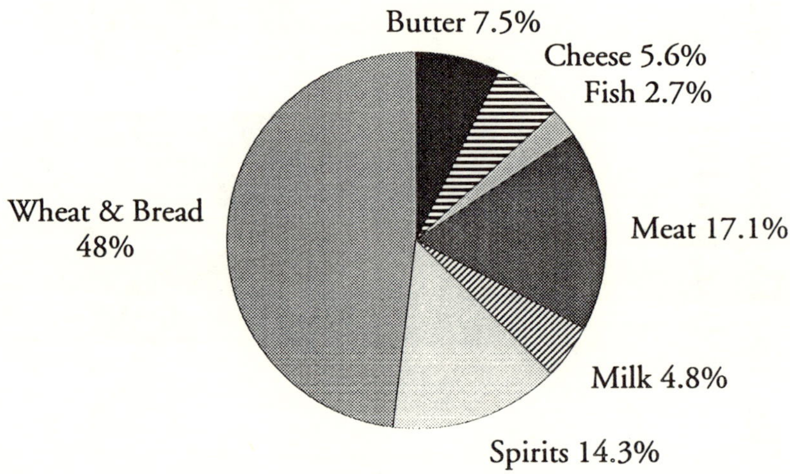

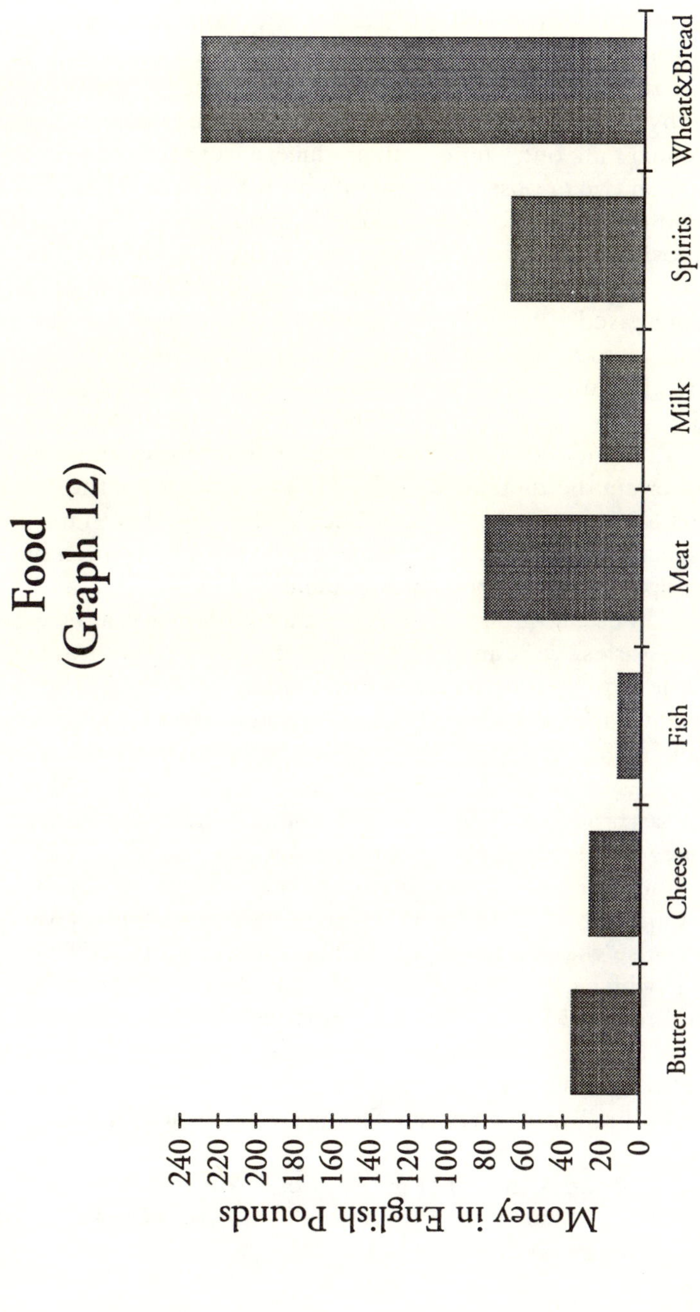
Food
(Graph 12)
Money in English Pounds
240
220
200
180
160
140
120
100
80
60
40
20
0
Butter
Cheese
Fish
Meat
Milk
Spirits
Wheat&Bread

young beadles. . . . "[4] The cost of nursing was not constant and varied with the number of children under the care of the hospital. This expenditure was very sensitive to the ages of the children; infants and toddlers required more care than older children. As mentioned, all of Christ's babies were cared for by wet nurses in their own homes. There is a physical limitation on how much milk one women can produce; a wet nurse could breast-feed no more than two or possibly three infants at one time. However, a single nurse tending to older children in the hospital could take care of two to three times as many. Therefore, the greater the number of small children, the greater the number of nurses were employed, and then the cost of nursing increased.

Payments to hospital staff other than nurses constituted only 9.4 percent of total regular expenditures (see graph 8). The average payment of staff expenses was £187 2s. 10d.[6] The largest payment, £303 1s. 11d., occurred in 1597 and the smallest payment, £1 4s., occurred in 1557 (see table 1). To ascertain the total impact of the cost of labor upon the hospital, the payments to nurses and staff have been added together. This combined labor discharge represented 34.8 percent of the regular payments (see graph 7). To supply the complete staffing needs of the hospital, both in-house and out-of-house, cost on the average nearly £700 per year (see graph 9).

"Necessaries" were an important part of annual expenditures and were, as the name implies, a group of assorted things that was felt to be indispensable. The average expenditure upon necessaries was the large sum of £468 1d. A total of £896.8049 was dispersed in 1589, which was the most money paid for necessaries; the smallest amount was £81.7909 in 1554 (see table 1). Necessaries accounted for 23.6 percent of the total and constituted the second-largest discharge of regular expenses (see graph 7). The bookkeeping decision to include it in the amorphous category of "necessaries" has no apparent logic; it may just be a convenient accounting category for items not fitting elsewhere in the budget. Clues can be assembled from the early records, in which each item purchased under this heading was individually listed. In June of 1553 the following items were listed as "necessaries": two pairs of shoes, three reimbursements to the matron, a "pole and the Carriage," a "sysed," a pulley and rope, two baskets, a pole for the wash house, a "qualle of ink," and a physician for the curing of sick children."[7] In June of 1554 these items were classed as "necessaries": milk, "soap and other necessaries," "shoes and other necessaries," "diverse necessaries," "sundry necessaries," "to Hopkyns the smith," "to Robert Cooke for making of certain apparel for the children," and "to John Hodgeson for his charges and in reward for going to Tylshelf."[8] By 1597–98, all that can be known about necessaries is what they were not. In that year, £364.8433 (£364 16s. 10d.) was not spent on board wages, pensions, nursing fees, officer's fees, "prestmoney" (loans), payments to and for Blackwell and Worsted Halls, fees for keeping the Book of Legacies, various obligations paid out of rent-producing properties, bread, various kinds of cloth, candles, wood, coal, butter and cheese, staff liveries, beer, fish, payments to the hospital's surgeon, three debt payments, beef & mutton, governors' dinners, the solicitor's fee, and extraordinary payments to the clerks of Blackwell Hall.[10] A necessary, it must be concluded, was whatever the treasurer or clerk decided it was.

In terms of the most important regular expenditures, food was the most important for the immediate comfort and care of the children, although it accounted for only 15.3 percent of the budget (see graph 8). The mean value of food was £303 6s. 3d., with the highest cost of £1010 16s. 1/4d. in 1555 and the lowest cost of £36 17s. 8d. occurring in 1564 (see table 1). Christ's Hospital bought dozens of items of food and drink for the consumption of the children. This included such diverse foodstuffs as raisins, pepper, and apple pies, as well as the staples of their diet: bread, beer, meat, cheese, and butter. To make it possible to comprehend the hundreds of categories of food discharges, food was aggregated under the broader headings of bread, milk, meat, butter, cheese, fish, and beer (see chart 5).[10]

Of course, certain foods played the greatest role in the ordinary diet of the children. Bread was the single most important item of food and was the staple of the children's diet, as it was of all Europeans at that time.[11] The combined outlay for both bread and wheat averaged £231 16s. 6d.; the largest payment was £3537 19s. in 1586 and the smallest payment of £335 17s. 3d. was made in 1593 (see table 1 and graph 12). Bread commanded by far the largest bite out of the budget, accounting for 48.0 percent or almost half of regular recorded food expenditures (see graph 11). It seems that the bread eaten at Christ's was not baked upon the premises but was prepared elsewhere and brought to the hospital: "That was agreed that the bread to serve this house shall be made hereafter at Bridewell, and to deliver 3 loaves for 2d. and any loaf to contain 20 ounces." [12]

Most entries of bread in the account books lack this wonderful detail about the weight of the bread and the price per loaf. They state simply the payment dispersed over a period of time, as this terse posting demonstrates: "paid to Clayton's widow and made even with her from the first day of the erection of this house which was the 11th of November/1552/ unto the last of June anno/1555/ as may appear . . . 280 Li."[13] It is once again illustrative of the nature of the documents that bread or wheat, which clearly must have been consumed in large quantities on a consistent basis, are lacking entries for the years 1552 and 1558 to 1576.

The purchase of meat accounted for 17.1 percent of regular recorded food items and was the second-largest expenditure (see graph 11). The average amount of money spent on meat was £82 7s. 6d. (see graph 12). The largest sum expended was £188 7s. 11d. in 1597 and the smallest sum expended was £3 18s. 9d. in 1557 (see table 1). It should be noted that average expenditure on meat is based upon only nine entries. At the Court of Governor's meeting on 20 of March 1591/92, the following entry indicates the careful scrutiny given to the children's diet.

> Francis Greene butcher is agreed with all to serve this house with beef and mutton, lamb or veal, the bones to be taken out of the beef, for one whole year to end at Shrovetide 1592 at 14d per stone one with another, and the same beef to be wholesome for the children bodies.[14]

A similar entry is made on 7 April, 1595 concerning William Clever. He was to be paid 15d. per stone.[15] This arrangement with the butcher demonstrates not only that the children enjoyed meat as a regular part of their diet, but also that some attempt was made to control the quality. Of course, having the bones removed would make the beef weigh less and would, therefore, be cheaper.

It is interesting that the only types of meat listed are beef, veal, lamb, and mutton; given the greater number of sheep than cattle in England, one would have expected less beef and more mutton. It is curious that neither pork nor fowl, both less expensive meats, is ever mentioned as being consumed in the hospital. However, there are expenditures for eggs: 12s. 6d. was "paid for 300 of eggs . . ."[16] It is difficult to chart the expenditures over time because there are only nine entries in which meat is entered as a separate item; meat consumption was probably higher. For example, the passage quoted above demonstrates that in 1592 Francis Greene acted as butcher to the hospital and specifies the price of the beef and mutton. However, in the Treasurer's Account Books, there is no record that meat was purchased in that year. Meat was probably purchased and listed under "necessaries."

Spirits—beer and small quantities of wine and ale—formed a regular provision of the children's diet and seems to have been the usual beverage at meals. Spirits averaged £69 7s. 8d. and constituted 14 percent of regular recorded food expenditures (see graphs 11 and 12). The largest sum spent on spirits was £313 1s. 11d. in 1597 and the smallest sum was £1 4s. in 1557 (see table 1).

Milk only constituted 4.8 percent of the recorded food expenses (see chart 6). There are only four entries for milk during the years 1553 to 1556, which means milk was probably entered in another category. The mean payment was £23 3s. 4d. The largest payment of £46 14s. 5d. was in 1554 and the smallest payment of £8 3s. was in 1556 (see table 1). A month's supply of milk was recorded on 28 September 1555; £1 2s. 6d. was spent on 108 gallons.

Milk was apparently only consumed as an ingredient in cooking or for its medicinal value. The hospital recorded regular purchases of both cheese and butter and is therefore doubtful that the milk purchased was used to produce any cheese and butter. Nor did milk form a regular part of the children's diet. Animal milk was not used, either, as a substitute for mother's milk; wet nurses were provided for babies. The belief was widespread that milk was "white blood" and that moral, intellectual, and emotional qualities could be transferred from women through breast milk to babies. "While the fetus exists in the womb it is nourished on blood, but at birth nature sends that blood to the breasts to be changed into milk."[17] "Animal milk was apparently not considered tolerable. Cow's milk is rarely mentioned and that of other beasts only as a horrid possibility since the child so nourished would resemble the source."[18] Because the consumption of animal milk was believed to result in undesirable animal characteristics being transmitted to people who drank it:

> Be sure that the wet nurse has plenty of milk because if she lacks it she may give the baby the milk of a goat or sheep or ass or some other animal because the child, boy or girl, nourished on animal milk doesn't have perfect wits like one fed on women's milk, but always looks stupid and vacant and not right in the head.[19]

Beer was considered a much more suitable drink for both adults and children and certainly was more available. The children of Christ's Hospital would have drunk beer in the same way that modern children consume milk, a fact that is very disturbing to modern adults. But Tudor adults would have been probably as appalled if you offered one of their children a glass of cow's milk.

Butter was also a regular part of the diet of the children, with the average discharge at £36 3s. 11d. (see graph 12). Butter was the fourth most expensive regularly recorded food item, accounting for 7.5 percent of the total (see graph 11). The largest amount spent on butter was £65 9s. 10d. in 1597 and the smallest amount was £9 8s. 10d. in 1553 (see table 1).

Cheese was a regular food purchase. The average expenditure upon cheese was £27 3s. 5d. and was 5.6 percent of the regular recorded food purchases (see graphs 11 and 12). Cheese was the fifth most expensive item of the children's fare. The largest outlay was in 1598, totaling £156 7s. 10d. The smallest outlay was in 1561 totaling £1 6s. (see table 1).

The least important food item in terms of mean payments was fish. Money spent upon fish only accounted for 2.7 percent of the total (see graph 11). The average outlay for fish was £12 11d.; the largest expenditure was £104 in 1579 and the smallest expenditure was 13s. 3d. in 1556 (see table 1 and graph 12). Fish must have been a regular feature of the children's diet, even though there are only twelve entries.[20] Although the limitations of the sources prevent a detailed quantitative analysis of the children's diet in terms of measuring the number of calories or grams of protein, fat, or carbohydrate, it is still possible to draw a general conclusion. The sheer variety of foodstuffs purchased by the hospital would indicate that the children were fed a diet that regularly included meat, butter, and cheese.

Pearce in his *Annals of Christ's Hospital*, cites a weekly menu for the children in 1678. Although this represents the diet of the hospital children in the seventeenth-century, and one must be wary about projecting such information backwards in time, it seems that the Tudor children were fed as well if not better.

> Sunday-noon – boiled beef and porridge with 5 oz of bread
> at night – roast mutton [The Public Supping]
> Monday-noon – water gruel with currants
> night – cheese
> Tuesday-noon – boiled beef
> night – cheese
> Wednesday-noon – Milk porridge bread & butter
> night – pudding pies without bread
> Thursday-noon – boiled beef
> night – cheese
> Friday-noon – milk porridge bread & butter
> night – pudding pies without bread
> Saturday – milk porridge with bread & butter at noon.
> night – cheese
> Every morning 2 1/2 oz. of bread and a sup of drink.
> 5 oz. of bread at every meal, dinner & supper.[22]

When visualizing English orphans, it is difficult not to call to mind the most famous orphan in English literature, Oliver Twist, and his struggle to survive in the infamous workhouse. There the children were each fed one little bowl of gruel as a meal, with a piece of bread thrown in on special occasions. "Oliver Twist and his companions suffered the tortures of slow starvation for three months," thereby prompting him the famous request, "Please, sir, I want some more."[22] As can be seen from the menu just cited, the children of Christ's Hospital were not left to eat gruel and water.

The money used to provide pensions to the sick and needy may constitute the most interesting category of budget expenditure. Pensions account for 12.6 percent of the regular expenditures and were the fourth most expensive budget item (see graph 7). The mean value of pensions paid out of the treasury of Christ's was £248 13s. 11d. (see graph 9) The largest drain of the hospital's money was in 1554, when pension payments totaled £868 19s. 7d. The smallest drain was in 1553, totaling £18 6d., a bookkeeping anomaly (see table 1).

Christ's Hospital from its foundation had assumed a wider responsibility than caring only for London's orphans. What is of interest here is not the numbers of pensioners and their pensions but the fact that the this orphanage gave money to people who were not children or parents. Why the governors of Christ's expanded their jurisdiction to include all sorts of poor and needy is never explained in the governors' court meeting records, but it is clear that Christ's Hospital acted as a central processing agency for the dispersal of poor relief throughout the City. The pension system of Christ's bears some similarity to the Social Security Administration in the United States, It provided money for the disabled, widows, orphans, the elderly, and the sick, but it had the advantage of being more flexible. As long as a person was needy but was not a vagabond, he or she could request assistance from the governors of Christ's.

To grant a pension to parents, the old, sick, and poor required the consent of the governors in a court meeting. Pensioners were obliged to produce a certificate from their parish vestries verifying that they were worthy of aid and had been a resident of London for three years. "And that no poor person be admitted to any pension, either to be paid in the parish or in this hospital, without the like certificate. . . ."[23]

As is explained in greater detail in chapter 6, a parent could be given assistance to help care for a child who was not an inmate of the hospital. "[T]here is granted unto John King toward the keeping of Jane his daughter of the age of 20 weeks 8d. weekly at the request of Master Castle of

Westminster."[24] Pensions were also assigned to people to keep children that were not their own: "Allowed unto Katherine Machan widow at London Stone toward the keeping of a woman child about the age of 4 years taken up by her in the streets 8d. weekly."[25]

The needy sick were also provided for also. "There was granted unto Robert Caffolde during the time of his sickness 6d. weekly to be paid in this house."[26] Illness of a spouse was a legitimate cause for obtaining relief. "There was also granted unto Robert Gates a capper toward the relief of his wife being sick & to his 4 children 6d. weekly."[27]

One could lay claim to a pension if one was disabled. "There was granted to John Hebbye soldier being blind toward his relief 8d. weekly."[28] The Senter couple was given a pension upon the condition that they would refrain from begging, and the fact that the wife was disabled surely weighed heavily in the decision of the governors. "Henry Senter and his wife with one leg 2 common beggars dwelling in Turnagaine Lane was forgiven the punishment for their beggary, and upon condition with their promise that here after they will labor and beg no more there is granted to every of them 4d. weekly."[29]

The elderly were also given pensions. "There was allowed unto John Cutberte aged and sick toward his relief 12d. weekly. . . ."[30] Also, women who were widows could petition for aid without necessarily having children. "There was also granted unto Elizabeth Coldwell widow toward her relief 6d. weekly."[31] Ex-officials could lay a claim to a pension from Christ's. "Unto John Broke late postmaster of Calais being poor, 6d. was allotted"[32] A weekly pension of 6d. was "Allowed unto William Borrough being bedridden late sexton of St. Sepulchre 6d weekly."[33] Pensions were reassigned due to the ineligibility or death of a former pensioner: "There is granted unto Agnes Dodd the pension which Elaine Giles deceased had which was 4d weekly."[34] Pensions were sometimes increased. "Allowed also unto Margery Walder lying bedridden beside the 8d. before granted other 8d. which is in the whole 16d. weekly."[35] Employees of Christ Hospital were granted pensions when they retired from service. "At this Court Margaret Backesteper sometime a nurse of this house was in consideration of her poor estate granted 6d. weekly to be paid in this house ye pleasure of ye governors."[36]

The last group of pensioners were the former inhabitants of the Savoy, a former leper hospital. As explained in the previous chapter, the lepers were given a pension, but this arrangement only lasted until 1557, at which time St. Thomas began to maintain its own accounts and took over these responsibilities. As of 9 of August 1557, Christ's Hospital was no longer responsible for the lazars' pensions. In total, this arrangement cost Christ's almost £312.[37]

Cloth and clothing accounted for 10.3 percent of the regular expenditure of the hospital and was the fifth-largest expenditure (see graph 7). The average expense for cloth and clothing was £203 3s. 6d., with the largest sum spent in 1583 (totaling £467 7 1/2d.) and the smallest sum spent in 1556 and (totaling a mere £15 11d.) (see table 1). Expenditure of money on cloth and clothing can be roughly divided into three groups: for cloth; for actual items of clothing; and for items necessary for either the dressing, weaving, sewing, or otherwise preparing of cloth or clothing for wear.[38] Some of this material was used in teaching the children the various crafts involved in processing cloth. For example, the children spun canvas, which was then made into shirts, smocks, and sheets.[39] Judging by the amount of clothing recorded, it would seem that the children also received a complete outfit of clothing at least once a year. The children were publicly visible due to their activities during City celebrations, especially the Spittle Sermon, and it must be presumed that on such important occasions they had to appear neat and tidy in respectable clothes. The children of Christ's Hospital were not clothed in rags but in a uniform that was worn daily and identified each child as belonging to Christ's Hospital.

From the fiscal year of 1567–68 until the fiscal year of 1581–82, the treasurer would offer a yearly summary of the amount of cloth and clothing purchased that year and how much was left. This special account was entered after the totals of charge and discharge and after the signatures of the auditors. For example, in the year 1566–67, it is recorded that northern plains [wool from northern England] went to make petticoats and that brown canvas was used for shirts and smocks. White cloth was turned into kerchiefs, biggens (caps, possibly night caps), and shirt bands (collars, similar to clerical collars). Hose was made out of wool and green cloth was used to make aprons. Blankets were made out of coarse white cloth and waistcoats were made out of white cotton. Shoes were, of course, made out of leather.[40]

Expenditures upon fuel comprised 3.1 percent of total regular expenditures (see graph 7). The average amount of money spent upon fuel totaled £60 14s. 6d., with the largest expenditure £162 17s. 6d., spent in 1556, and the smallest expenditure £3 6s., spent in 1558 (see table 1 and graph 9). Coal was the main heating source used by the hospital. The average payment for coal amounted to £39 14s. 6d. The largest sum dispersed upon coal was £136 19s. 9d. in 1556, and the smallest sum was £3.3000 6s. in 1558 (see table 1). The other type of fuel consumed by Christ's was billets, which were simply wood. Coal was the more important fuel source and accounted for almost two-thirds of the total cost of fuel. Because of the decreasing supply of wood, there was an increasing demand for coal by the hospital and the rest of London. By the mid-seventeenth century, the vast importation of coal into London from Newcastle would cause a serious problem of air pollution.[41]

The smallest item of regular expenditure was that spent on candles; this accounted for only 0.4 percent of the total regular expenditures (see graph 7). The mean value of money spent on candles was £8 5s. 4d., with the largest amount spent in 1598 (totaling £19 9s. 4d.) and the smallest amount spent in 1574, totaling £1 4s. (see tables 1 and 9).[42] The hospital purchased wick candles, watch candles, and cotton candles, though the distinction between these different varieties is not evident. Watch candles were more expensive, costing in 1573 2s. 10d. a dozen while wick candles cost 2s. 6d. a dozen in the same year; cotton candles were not purchased regularly. Watching candles may have been used as night lights for the various parts of the hospital. It would seem that Christ's usually bought their candles, but in 1566 and 1567 tallow was bought instead and made into candles. The sum of £6 10s. 8d. was paid to "Master Broke agent to the worshipful Company of Russia for 7 100th weight of Moscow tallow bought of him the 27th day of September 1567 at 17s. 8d. the 100th."[43] The preceding year Christ's had purchased not only tallow from the Muscovy Company but flax as well. The reason for the exotic purchase of Russian tallow may be explained by the fact that Sir William Chester, "one of the earliest benefactors of Christ's Hospital[,] . . . was governor of the Muscovy Company."[45]

In addition to the regular expenses detailed above, Christ's spent money on items and services that were needed on an occasional basis. The price of legal assistance was such a semiregular expense. The cost rose as time progressed, which was to be expected as gifts of land and money to the hospital inevitably involved legal disputes over the provisions and intentions of a benefactor. The mean value of legal expenses was £22 8s. 5d. Christ's spent the most on its legal affairs in 1590—£93 3s. 4d.—and the least in 1576, 10s. (see table 1).

The hospital retained its own solicitor; £26 6s. 8d. was "Paid to Master Wright Solicitor for this house for his year's fee ended at Michaelmas Last."[45] However, at various points in time the cost of extraordinary legal help accounted for a rather hefty sum of money. The amount of £36 10s. was paid to Mr. Wright "to follow the Suit in Law against Master Kempe concerning Master Walter's legacy to the hospitals."[46]

> 50s. was paid for the defense of John Vandernot in law, for withholding from this house a certain plot called the porter's lodge on the one side of the west door of the great cloister, and of a school house on the other side of the same cloister, which at the lease the same Vandernot clearly released and resigned to the use of this house.[47]

Three pounds was "Paid for council & other charges about ye assurance making to Christ's Hospital from ye right worshipful Sir Thomas Ramsey knight & alderman of London and Dame Marie his wife of their gift, viz, of ye priory of Beerden and parsonage of Oaueringe."[48] As part of the £3 spent upon securing undisputed ownership of the property bequeathed by Sir Thomas Ramsay, £1 was given

> To Master Weekes and Master Owen at their going to Islington with the Governors to the Queen's Majesty's Solicitor, to confer with him in this cause, and to have his opinion of our Corporation for the safer holding of the said gift, Master Solicitor being not then at home.[49]

Though the majority of legal disputes were over property, other disagreements could arise from time to time. At least once, the governors charged a man with slander. The large sum of £8 9s. was "Paid for charges in law in the suit of John Selby woodmonger, for certain slanderous and reproachful speeches by him spoken and uttered against ye Treasurer and Governors of this house."[50]

Routine transfers of property involved fees to register ownership, as shown by the £2 10s. 4d. dispensed "To the Clerk of Enrollments, and for ye Master of the Rolls fee for the enrollment in ye Chancery of the Indenture of Bargain and sale from Sir Thomas Ramsey the 28 of March, 1584. . . ."[51] A £1 charge was paid to the "prerogative court" every year "To William Boddie one of Master Argell's clerk for this year's fee for keeping of a Register of the Legacies given to this hospital. . . ."[52]

Given the litigious nature of Tudor society, it would have been expected that Christ's Hospital would have expended more funds upon legal affairs, especially since it was located in London, which was the center of the English judicial system and where it was relatively easy to take a dispute to court for resolution. Lawrence Stone describes litigation as "the most popular of indoor sports" for the aristocracy and that would have also held true for other landlords, even hospitals.[53] However, on average, Christ's paid more of its income for butter and cheese than it did for lawyers or lawsuits.

Medical costs have also been classified as a semiregular expense. For the period of time covered by this study there were only eight medically related expenditures totaling £30.2165. It is probable that the category of "necessaries" covered most medical expenses. However, the account books record the following entries for various medical expenses. Seven shillings was "paid for the healing of 4 children's head."[54] The amount of 20d. was "paid the 14th of April to Trinian Carsley for the healing of a young child diseased with the pox"[55] and 12d. was "paid also in reward to a woman of Richmond for curing of a child's mouth. . . ."[56]

Exclusive of the previous medical accounting were the entries for the "diet of the sick children." Food for sick children would have been intended to serve as medicine rather than as plain nourishment. In the first week of October, 24s. 10d. was "paid for the diet of sick children."[57] The amount of £5 10s. was "paid to the Matron the 8 day of April for the diet of 100 sick children. . . ."[58] Four shillings was "paid for 2 stand of ale for sick children. . . ."[59] Food, in the predetermined amounts and combinations, comprised an important part of any medical treatment in this period.

Although routine illnesses were attended to by the staff nurses and afflicted children were confined in the sick ward, outside professional medical care was sometimes needed. Five pounds was "Paid to Master Martine surgeon to this house for a benevolence. . . ."[60] Christ's dispersed 40s. in 1553 "to a foreign physician for the healing of diverse sick and lame children. . . ."[61]

The cost of maintaining the buildings and grounds of the hospital decreased after the initial outlay involved in converting the Greyfriars Monastery to an orphanage. In 1552 and 1553 £326 12s. 1d. was invested in the conversion of the old monastery into the new hospital. However, on average, Christ's spent £25 17s. 5d. for associated building and maintenance costs; the largest sum was in 1553, totaling £220 11s., and the smallest sum was in 1595, totaling 2s. 10d. (see table 1). Repairs, by their very nature, are unpredictable and highly irregular in nature. Christ's Hospital was not only responsible for keeping its own property in good repair but also its rental properties, as explained in chapter 3. The hospital employed, at various times, a variety of laborers and craftsmen. These included bricklayers, blacksmiths, plumbers, plasterers, pavers, carpenters, painters, and tilers. Eight pounds was paid "To John Band carpenter for timber and setting up the Scaffold in Christ's Church for the children to set upon" while attending their parish church.[62] In 1586 £1 9s. 6d. was "Paid, for painting [the] Counting house which was new made. . . ."[63] In the fiscal year 1580–81, £340 was allocated "for the new building and full finishing of five new tenements in the round Woolstaple at Westminster. . . ."[64]

Keeping the plumbing in good working order was not inexpensive. The large expenditure in 1555 of 28s. 2d. was "paid for works done by the plumber for the amendment of the water pipes and bringing home again the water to Christ's Hospital. . . ."[65] In 1563 the hospital paid £19 7d. for "reparations at the conduit head."[66] The amount of £58 6s. 5d. was laid out in 1564 to go to "The new making of the great cistern for the common conduit with 5 cisterns & a pump for the wash house with the house on the same cistern and conveying water in to ye sick ward. . . ."[67] In 1577 19s. 6d. was the outlay "To the plumber for reparations of the water pipes and the conduit heads belonging to this hospital. . . ."[68]

An additional outlay of £64 6s. 2d. was needed the following year to pay plumbers, bricklayers, masons, carpenters, and laborers for "Reparations at the conduit heads. . . ."[69] In 1597, the large amount of £79 15s. 5d. was dispersed to pay for the lead needed "for the amending of the pipes belonging to this house" and for plumbers and laborers to fix the plumbing.[70]

The particular maintenance needs of the hospital's sick ward involved irregular outlays. A total of £5 2s. 4d. was spent "for rafters, quarters and penthouse boards and for 2 men's wages for 12 days about weather boarding in the garden and in mending of bedsteads in the sickward. . . . "[71] In 1566 £6 was paid to "William Ape plumber for a cistern of lead in the sickward and for other work done there. . . ."[72] In 1572 £125 2s. 3d. was allocated for the timber, tile, nails, pipes, and labor needed "in building of the new sick ward,"[73]

In 1577 it was decided to build a new countinghouse, which cost £117 14s. 4 1/2d. A further 40s. was spent "for 5 yards of green cloth for a carpet at 8s the yard, for the new counting house."[74] In 1581 £17 1s. 10d. was expended for "reparations & for a new gallery. . . ."[75]

Another major expense was involved in building and maintaining the structures around St. Mary Spittle, which was the site of the annual Spittle Sermon. This part of the Easter celebration was the biggest festival of the calendar year at which the children sang. The purpose of the Spittle Sermon was not merely to give the children religious instruction through a good Easter sermon but to provide the opportunity for the citizens of London to observe the children of Christ's Hospital, thereby publicizing the hospital (which might elicit further donations). In his diary, Henry Machin records that he witnessed "a goodly sermon" at the Spittle on 19 April 1557. The event was impressive:

> [T]here was my Lord Mayor and 13 aldermen beside my Lord Mayor . . . and all the masters of the hospital . . . and all the children of the hospital in blue garments both at men children and women children, that be kept with certain lands and the charity of the nobility of London. . . .[76]

It was also important that the staff of Christ's looked like they had decent attire, and £6 10s. 6d. was "Paid to the nurses and beadles for their liveries always against Easter to attend upon the governors and children. . . ."[77] To insure the comfort of the governors and children and also to save some money, £140 was

> Paid to Master Willford chamberlain of London for charges in building a house in St. Marie Spittle for ye Governors and the children to sit and hear the sermons there yearly preached in the Easter holy days, by the hands of Mistress Alice Elkine, the sum of one hundred & forty pounds – by the building of which house there is yearly saved, 7Li, or 8Li, at the least, by setting up, & taking down a scaffold which was there set up. . . . [78]

In addition to the £140 a further sum of £6 16s. was dispensed that same year "Paid to Freesingfield painter for work done upon the said house, beautifying and painting of sundry arms, and other things. . . ."[79] A total of £18 4s. 3d. was given "To the plumber for his bill for lead and work done about the new building at St. Mary Spittle. . ."[80] Further work was done in the following year, 1595, by "William Highwaie bricklayer for work done at St. Mary Spittle. . . " He received £6 10s. for his efforts.[81] An old tent that once provided cover for the children and governors, and had been rendered superfluous by the building of permanent structures, was recycled. "[T]hat was ordered that ye said tent shall be cut & made into cases for ye children's beds & to be filled with straw for that ye straw of ye children's beds lying loose as that now doth is troublesome to ye nurses and wards in ye making of ye beds."[82] It also illustrates that the children had real beds that were made up on a regular basis and that the governors were attentive to the complaints of their staff. Certainly the governors thought that the Spittle Sermon was important enough to warrant the expenditure of large sums of money from time to time.

Some of the expenditures made by the treasurer were a requirement of a legacy or bequest to the hospital. An example of a regular payment as part of a conditional gift was the requirement to cover the costs of annual repairs to the conduit heads on Sir Martin Bowes's gift of land. Conduit heads were an essential part of the water supply and regular inspection was necessary to ensure that the pipes were not damaged or blocked. If they were not annually visited by the Lord Mayor, presumably for the purpose of inspection, then a fine had to be paid to the Goldsmiths. (Sir Martin Bowes had himself been a goldsmith.) Hence we read that £4 was paid "To the Company of Goldsmiths, for that ye Lord Mayor did not visit the conduit heads, this year."[83] And £6 13s. 4d. was paid "To the Chamber of London, towards the repairing of the conduit heads of this city for, 1 year ended at Michaelmas."[84] Another example of a conditional payment is the £8 paid out of the income from Castell's gift of land "To the poor of St. Margaret in Westminster due always in the beginning of December before Christmas."[85]

Rewards were disbursements of money to persons for unusual service and formed a diversified category of outlay for the hospital. Thus 12s. 2d.was "paid in reward to John Hodgeson at two several times going into the country to remove certain children that were not well used, and for the carriage of the same from one place to an other. . . ."[86] Also listed as a reward was the 9s. "paid to John Vandernot for certain chalk found in the schoolhouse, and for a lock that was upon the door. . . ."[87] In another example, £1 was settled upon "William Braiford servant unto Sir Martin Bowes for engrossing of the writing of Sir Martin's gift to this house. . . ."[88]

Benevolences were not only a source of income for Christ's but also a category of expenditure. This designation covered an assortment of payments. For example, the cost of maintaining scholars at Cambridge and Oxford universities was classed as a "benevolence." One pound was paid "To Thomas Austen the 5th of February, a scholar of Oxenford . . . "[89] and another £1 was paid "To John Duffeild saddler towards ye helping of his son William at the University who was sometime one of the poor children of this hospital. . . ."[90] Another type of benevolence, which may have been a legal settlement, was the £30 "Given and paid to Henry Hampcots gentleman in full satisfaction of a claim made by him of land in Westham being the gift of Mr. Hamon Hampcots. . . ."[91] Also classified as a benevolence was the £10 paid "To, George Howe & Richard Wood painters for a piece of work painted which hangeth at the south end of the great hall. . . ."[92] Benevolence could also be used to dismiss bad debts, as was the case with the £8 19s. owed by Giles Strother: "was forgiven him his old debt. . . ."[93]

Annuities, like benevolences, were not only a form of income but a category of expenditure. Eight pounds was paid "To, John Lawrence of Hackney and Elizabeth his wife for this year's annuity given them, during their natural lives, in consideration of yielding up the lease of a house with ye fee simple of another in Tuttle street at Westminster."[94]

Other irregular payments related directly to the hospital's function as a school. Writing paper, pens, inkhorns, and books were purchased for the children to facilitate their studies. The substantial sum of £12 15s. 8d. was allotted with the notation "Books paid for to Master Norton for 2 year's last past, for ye children of this house. . . ."[95] The Tudor version of alphabet blocks were provided by Christ's to help in the children's learning and 2s. 8d. was "paid for one hundred alphabets upon boards."[96] The substantial sum of £8 was used to purchase "32 reams of paper at 5s per reams."[97]

As explained in the previous chapter, Christ's Hospital received, as a major source of income, money from both Blackwell and Worsted Halls, with the provision that the hospital pay the operating expenses of these institutions. The average cost of operating Blackwell Hall was £61 7s. 9 1/2d. with the cost as high as £182 15s. 11d. in 1589 and as low as £46 9s. 7d. in 1580 (see table 1). The outlay for the operation of Blackwell Hall comprised cash payments for officers' fees, wages, rents, and other assorted expenses.[98] Additional items of cost to keep Blackwell running were recorded. Thus £2 15s. 2d. was allocated for cleaning the privy in Blackwell Hall: "Paid to Edward Downs nightman for the making clean a privy taking out thereof 28 tons of filth," a task comparable to the cleaning of the Augean Stables.[99] The sum of £25 14s. 6d. was paid for what was described as simply "reparations done upon Blackwell Hall. . . ."[100]

Costs for operating Worsted Hall averaged a mere £18 8s. 8d.; the largest outlay was £122 19s. 6d. in 1580 and the smallest was the 4s. paid in both 1583 and in 1584 (see table 1).[101]

Additional occasional expenditures give an insight into the varied activities that Christ's Hospital assumed in its role as a charitable institution, though, in themselves, they hold little significance. Sixpence was "paid for a corked shoe for a lame wench. . . ."[102] Transportation costs were paid not only for goods for the hospital but for the governors as well. Twelve shillings was "Paid for boat hire to and from Westminster to peruse the writings of Master Castell's lands in the hands of Samuel Garsh. . . And to and from the Lord Chancellors;[103] . . . 8d. was paid for 2 sheep skins to make the boys of the kitchen jerkins."[104] Sixpence was "paid to the matron for washing the linen."[105] Seven pence was an "Item given for the burying of a poor man."[106]

Two shillings was an "Item given to Thomas Lucas for cleansing of the Jaques [toilet]."[107] Sixpence was "paid for mending of a water tankard" and 5s. 2d. was "paid for apple pies for Friday dinner." [109] The sum of 40s. 8d. was "paid for the charge of the dinner of election," the annual dinner given on the day of election of the new governors for the hospital.[110] Three shillings was "paid for printing of certain precepts."[111] Eighteen pence was "paid for a tiler & labourer one day."[112] Twenty-six shillings, eight pence was "paid to John Bonde for making of a cross in the churchyard and for stuff."[113] Sixteen pence was "paid for cleansing the kitchen roof."[114] Eight pence was "paid for grinding of kitchen knives"[115] and 10d. was "paid for sponge for the well."[116] Eighteen pence was "paid for the carriage of a poor woman that was lunatic to Bedlem."[117] Five shillings was used to purchase "certain hooks for the slaughter house."[118] The £2 16s. 4d. paid for a new kettle was quite a deal, because the purchase price was decreased in consideration for "the exchange of an old kettle for the washhouse. . . ."[119]

When one considers the hundreds of items purchased by the hospital for the comfort and care of the children, an obvious question presents itself: Why did not the governors cut back radically on expenditures when in fiscal crisis? Or put more simply, why was the children's care so good? It does not seem to have entered into the economic considerations of the governors to reduce the costs of maintaining the hospital by decreasing the quality of the diet or the clothes of the children. By and large this must be a reflection of the perceptions and attitudes of the governors; they decided what was the appropriate food for the children based upon what they themselves ate.

John Howes indicates that the governors treated the children of Christ's Hospital as if they were their own.

> They are bound to be as careful for the virtuous bringing up of these children as well in good qualities apt & fit for children as if they wear there own having in mind that their own children their sons or daughters children may be relieved by that which now they relieve others, which being themselves but stewards for the goods of the world are mutable & God raiseth and God pulleth down.[120]

The governors, then, assumed a responsibility toward the children under their care that extended far beyond providing the minimum requirements for mere survival. "[T]hey that abide in the shelter of Christ's Hospital and share the king's bounty shall have their minds and hearts fed, as well as their baser parts."[121] The children were not fed gruel and water but a diet that included meat and dairy products. The children of Christ's were not clothed in rags but in clothes made out of good-quality cloth. Although they wore special clothes that identified them as Christ's Hospital children, it was not to instill shame but pride. The governors also believed that schooling was a crucial part of the care they provided. These children seem to have been provided with the basics of life in sufficient quantity and quality to give them a fighting chance of arriving at a healthy, productive adulthood.

5
Governors and Guardians

> I am persuaded that the Governors of all the Hospitals as well of Bridewell as of the rest are men that fear God & of so good conscience that they would not for any worldly wealth be touched with any corruption or gain in ministering of Justice. . . .
>
> —John Howes (1587)

> I here see this merciful work towards the poor; whom I must, in the midst of my royalty, needs remember.
>
> —Queen Elizabeth I (1559)

The men who served in the capacity of governor to the four hospitals of London were among the leading citizens of London (see Appendix B). These were the same men who filled various offices for the City and the guilds, and for their parishes. To be a governor of a hospital was an extension of a general sense of civic responsibility. Governors were not paid for their time and services, but their expertise was freely given first as an obligation to their community and second as a Christian imperative to aid those less fortunate. It would be a mistake to ascribe a purely secular motive to the labors of the governors. These men saw their service to their fellow man as an important aspect of their Christianity; if this duty was not performed properly, the governors believed that they would be called to account before God for their actions.

> [E]very of you that ye here promise before God and us this assembly of your fellow governors faithful to travail in this your charge be diligently and whol somely provided for as ye will answer before God at the hour and time when you and we shall stand before him to render an account of our doings, and you promising this to do shall be now admitted into this company and fellowship.[1]

This declaration was to be administered to the "new governors always the Monday following their election. . . ."[2]

The governors did not merely sit occasionally at breakfast meetings upon the boards of these charitable organizations and give nods of approval to policy to be executed by salaried employees. The governors were responsible for the day-to-day running of the hospitals. The governors both decided upon and implemented policies that involved serious obligations. These men had also served the City in other capacities and they brought that experience to their hospital duties. It seems that the governors did not distinguish one office from other; on the court days they did not just act as governors of a royal hospital but also as aldermen, company wardens, and parish officials. They were not just hospital governors but also representatives of the Corporation of London.

The hospitals, almost from their beginnings, were intricately woven into the institutional fabric of the City. The governorships were an important part of the greater civic responsibility of administering the City offices.

> Governor of one of the four hospitals was the first important civic office. In 1559 there were 48 governors, 12 aldermen and 36 common councilmen; in 1599 there were 176 governors, 24 aldermen and 152 councilmen. Other offices or duties might be assumed around the same time as hospital governor, though none had the same prestige.[3]

To fill the position as a governor took a good deal of time and work; the individual had to attend weekly court meetings and be willing to serve additionally on various ad hoc committees. For example on 5 April 1560

> there were also appointed to have the onsight and to peruse the book of legacies certain Governors whose names here after are expressed: Master Mathews, Master Springham, Master Grafton, Master Ducket, Master Beswicke, Master Lamberte, Master Hulson, Master Barnham.[4]

On the same date, Heton, Quarles, and Grafton were selected to examine "the ordinary collection that cometh to Christ's Hospital, and to devise some mean[s] to increase the same which [was] great decayed."[5]

The vast majority of governors were members of the twelve great guilds of London. An examination of Appendix B, which details the years of governorships for the four hospitals, illustrates overwhelming membership in "the twelve." However, not all the great guilds were equally represented. Most of the governors belonged to the mercers, grocers, drapers, skinners, merchant tailors, clothworkers, and haberdashers. The salters, ironmongers, vintners, fishmongers, and goldsmiths were underrepresented, a circumstance that parallels the representation of the guilds in the office of Lord Mayor.

> In addition to holding the office of alderman the aspirant must also be a member of one of the twelve leading companies. And, though each of these companies nominally had a right equal to every other one, in the period of years covered by the Tudor rule 24 per cent of the mayors were mercers, while not quite 2 per cent were vintners.[6]

An illustration of the support given to the royal hospitals by the City leadership is the fact that the vast majority of the Lord Mayors served as governors of one or more of them. Of the sixty-three Lord Mayors of London starting with Martin Bowes (1545–46) and ending with James Pemberton (1611–12), all but two had served the hospitals as governors. The exceptions were John Watts (1606–7) and Robert Lee (1602–3).[7] Of those sixty-one Lord Mayors who did serve as governors, twenty-seven served as governors of Christ Hospital, which is 43.8 percent (see Appendix B).[8]

The governors did not normally serve as governors for only one hospital; it was not unusual for a governor to use his talents and ambition for the benefit of more than one. Some of the governors of Christ's went on to perform the duties of president and treasurer for the other hospitals. Edmund Style, who was governor of Christ's in 1556–57, also officiated as a treasurer of St. Barts in 1557–58, in addition to being a governor of that hospital. Sir Richard Saltenstall, a skinner, was a sheriff in 1588–89 and Lord Mayor in 1597–98, an M.P. for London in 1586–87, a governor of the Merchant Adventurers, and collector of customs for London. He became the treasurer for St. Thomas before becoming a governor of Christ's in 1591–92 and was auditor general from 1583–84 until 1586–87. Although serving as president of St. Thomas Hospital, Sir John Rivers, grocer, was first a governor of Christ's, starting in 1570–71; he was a sheriff in 1565–66 and Lord Mayor in 1573–74. Thomas Gardener, goldsmith, was a governor of Christ's from 1561–62 until 1562–63, and later the treasurer of Bridewell, starting in 1573–74. Sir Lionel Ducket, mercer, was governor of the orphanage from 1557–58 until 1559–60, later officiating as president of St. Thomas in the fiscal year of 1573–74. In addition to the presidency of St. Thomas, Ducket assumed the presidency of Bridewell from 1580–81 until 1585–86. Ducket was sheriff in 1564–65 and Lord Mayor in 1572–73. Sir Alexander Avenon, ironmonger, who held the offices of sheriff in 1561–62 and Lord Mayor in

1569–70, was also president of Bridewell from 1573–74 until 1580–81; he was president of St. Thomas for two years, from 1571–72 until 1572–73. In addition to the presidency of these two hospitals, Avenon was a governor of Christ's from 1563–64 until 1567–68.[9]

The procedure to elect the presidents of the four hospitals is not clear. The presidency seems to have fallen upon the most senior citizen who had already served as sheriff and Lord Mayor.

> Succession to presidencies of the four hospitals did not at first follow any discernible order. The court apparently felt that all senior aldermen, and some juniors, should have the leadership. There was frequent shuffling of men from one position to another in order to give as many aldermen as possible some responsibility. After about the middle of the 1570s, however, procedures began to crystallize. Thereafter succession to a presidency was usually to the most senior of those beyond the chair who had not yet held such a position. Each succeeding presidency then went to a man the junior of his predecessor.[10]

Who were these governors and what was their influence upon the maintenance and growth of the hospital? It would be difficult to list the hundreds of men who served as governors of the hospital. The intent in this chapter is to examine the major "movers and shakers" of the hospital, namely the governors who also served as its presidents and its treasurers.

According to the records of Christ's and the City, the presidents of Christ's during the years of this study were Sir Thomas Offley (1559), Sir Thomas Ramsay (1582), Sir Wolstan Dixie (1590), and Sir Richard Martin (1594). There is some confusion over the presidency of Christ's, due mostly to the lack of information before 1559, the year that Christ's began to identify presidents in its Minutes of the Court of Governors. E. H. Pearce, in his book *Annals of Christ's Hospital*, lists the following men as presidents of the orphanage: Sir George Barnes, 1553; Sir Martin Bowes, 1556; Sir Andrew Judd, 1556; Sir Thomas Offley, 1559; Sir Thomas White, 1563; Sir Thomas Ramsey, 1582; Sir Wolstan Dixie, 1590; and Sir Richard Martin, 1593.[11] Beaven, in his *Aldermen of London*, states that Pearce's dating of the presidency of Christ's is not, in all cases, accurate. He asserts that in his own list "The dates for such appointments . . . have been verified in every instance by reference to the Court Books, and in the few early cases where these fail to supply them, to the City records."[12] Beaven doesn't acknowledge the presidency of Andrew Judd, Thomas White, or Martin Bowes. The other records of the hospital also fail to reveal conclusive dating for the

Presidents of Christ's Hospital

Name	*Guild*	*Alderman*	*Master/ Warden*	*Sheriff*	*Lord Mayor*	*Birthplace*	*Other Hosp. Service*	*Other*
Offley (1599–63)	Merchant Tailor	Portsoken (1549–50) Aldgate (1550–82)	1547–48	1553–54	1556–57	Stafford	Surveyer General (1567–72) Comptroller General (1572–82)	
Ramsey (1582–90)	Grocer	Cheap (1566–88) Cornhill (1588–90)		1567–68	1577–78	Unknown	Surveyor General (1586–90) Governor-St. Bart's (1559–61)	
Dixie (1582–90)	Skinner	Broad St. (1586, 1588)	1573, 1576	1575–76	1585–86 1580, 1583	Catworth Huntingdon Shire		
Martin (1593–1602)	Goldsmith	Farringdon Within (1578–98) Bread St. (1598–1602)		1581–82	1589 & 1594	Unknown	Comptroller General (1594–1602) Governor–St. Bart's (1564–66)	Warden of the Mint (1559–95) Master of the Mint (1580–1617)

presidency in its early years. A list found in the Book of Legacies prepared by John Hawes, treasurer of Christ's in 1632, has the presidents as follows: Sir George Barnes,1553; Sir Thomas Offley, 1559; Sir Thomas Ramsey, 1582; Sir Wolston Dixie, 1590; and Sir Richard Martin, 1593/94. In short, Pearce's and Hawes's lists must be discounted, leaving Offley, Ramsey, Dixie, and Martin as the only certain presidents of the hospital in the sixteenth century.

These men had certain things in common. All of the presidents served as aldermen, sheriffs, and Lord Mayors. Furthermore, most of the presidents were masters of their guilds, non-native Londoners, and served as governors of the other three royal hospitals.

The aldermen were an important and indispensable body of citizens, and their duties were wide-ranging. There were a total of twenty-six aldermen, one for each ward of the City. There was no time limit on how long they could serve; some would remain aldermen for decades. An alderman could represent more than one ward in his career but not at the same time. Aldermen were supposed to reside within their wards.

> According to the act of common council passed in Henry IV's reign, the aldermen were required to live in the wards they represented. . . . It would seem then, that attempts were made by the city to compel the residence of the alderman in the ward which he represented, but that the attempts were not crowned with success, and that in some cases the alderman did not actually live with in the city's limits.[13]

The aldermen were chiefly responsible for upholding the law and maintaining order in their wards. "Within his own ward, he carried a special responsibility; he would have to be well acquainted with the householder, preside over the ward moot, and see to the organization of the watch."[14] The other important duty of aldermen was to sit in

> the Court of Aldermen, whose twenty-six members each represented one of the wards of the City. Over their meetings there presided the Mayor. . . . The far-reaching responsibilities of the Court of Aldermen included the maintenance of the privileges of the City and the enforcement of public order. From its seat at the Guildhall, this body controlled a complex series of institutions. . . . The Lord Mayor and Aldermen also sat as a law court to hear actions brought by citizens. . . . In addition, the alderman might well find himself engaged at a high political level, perhaps representing the City before the Privy Council, and attending at the royal court.[15]

Sir Thomas Offley represented two wards as alderman: Portsoken (1549–50) and Aldgate (1550–82).[16] Sir Thomas Ramsey represented the ward of Cheap from 1566 until 1588 and the ward of Cornhill from 1588 until 1590, the year of his death.[17] Sir Wolstan Dixie was alderman from Broad Street Ward from 1574 to 1593 and alderman from Bassishaw Ward from 1593 to 1594.[18] Sir Richard Martin, the last sixteenth-century president of Christ's, served as alderman from Aldersgate from 1579 to 1588 and from Cheap from 1588 to 1589.[19]

All the presidents served the City as sheriffs. The office of sheriff was the second most important position in London; it required two leading citizens to serve one term of a year's duration.

> Two sheriffs were chosen annually by Congregation for one year only. Though one was elected for the county of Middlesex, the other for the City of London, their jurisdictions had overlapped for centuries. By the time they began serving their shrieval years, most Elizabethans were already aldermen, and their succession to the shrievalty followed by order of seniority on the Court of Aldermen.[20]

Turning again to the list of Christ's presidents, Offley was sheriff in 1553–54 with Sir William Huet, who was a president of St. Thomas Hospital. Ramsey was sheriff in the administrative year of 1567–68, serving with Sir John Langley. Dixie was elected as a sheriff in 1575–76 along with Edward Osborne, who was president of St. Thomas Hospital from 1586 to 1592. Richard Martin was one of the sheriffs in 1581–82, having served with Sir William Webbe.[21]

Lord Mayor was the highest office in London. The Lord Mayor was elected in September for a single annual term. The man who became Lord Mayor was usually the most senior alderman who had served as sheriff but had not yet served as Lord Mayor. "The election of the mayor was held annually in the Guildhall. Prior to 1546 the elections took place on St. Edward's Day (October 13), but on account of the expenses of the feasts, an act of common council of that year changed the date to Michaelmas, on which day the sheriffs took their oaths."[22] The major requirement of the office of Lord Mayor of London was service as an "alderman for a considerable length of time. . . . In addition to holding the office of alderman the aspirant [also had to] be a member of one of the twelve leading companies."[23] A prospective Lord Mayor had to have been sheriff. And lastly, the candidate had to be wealthy, because the expenses required to maintain the position as the leading citizen of the leading city of the realm necessitated a large purse.

> Besides the great feast which he was compelled to give on the day he was sworn into office, the mayor was supposed to give additional banquets at various seasons of the year. Moreover, he was expected to entertain any foreigner of rank, or any official of the English crown who happened to visit London.[24]

As part of the recognition by the Crown of the difficult and critical duties performed by Lord Mayors, they were usually knighted during their term.

The duties of the Lord Mayor were manifold. He remained as one of the twenty-six alderman representing the wards into which the City was administratively divided, and he still had to perform his aldermanic obligations.[25] Part of the mayor's job was to supervise some aspects of the City's food supply. "As clerk of the market, the mayor regulated the prices of food and the assize of bread and beer, and inspected the weights and measures used in the city. When the prices of wheat rose or fell, the mayor ordered a corresponding change in the size of the loaf of bread."[26] The mayor was also responsible for executing health regulations. Severe measures were mandated when the City was afflicted with the plague, which was endemic until 1665. "One of the most important of his duties regarding the welfare of the metropolis was the mayor's oversight of the public health. As a health officer he had charge of the sanitary conditions of the houses, streets and lanes."[27] Settling disputes, whether they involved individuals, companies, or parishes,[28] constituted another aspect of the Lord Mayor's job. He either presided over the Court of Aldermen or settled disputes under his own authority. Additionally, he was required to raise soldiers in time of national need.

> As lord lieutenant of the city of London, the mayor received a commission for the mustering and training of troops at times when the realm was in need of armed forces. His commission was usually sent at the same time as those of the lords lieutenants of the counties. In this capacity it was his duty to ascertain the number of able-bodied men and the quantity of arms that the city could furnish, to oversee the training of the men. . . . [29]

When the monarch needed to raise money by loans, the mayor was responsible for collecting the funds from among his citizens. "Any information which the crown officials were desirous of having imparted to the companies was sent first to the Lord Mayor."[30] The mayor also held responsibility for all City institutions, including prisons and the hospitals: "After the dissolution of the monasteries the hospitals of the city were placed in charge of the mayor."[31] Therefore, the Lord Mayor was ultimately accountable for the operations of all the royal hospitals, including Christ's Hospital, and could overturn decisions made by their governors, although this was seldom done. In short, the Lord Mayor was the primary executive officer for London and was its chief representative and spokesman, especially when interacting with the Crown or the Privy Council.

Sir Thomas Offley was Lord Mayor in 1556–57. Sir Thomas Ramsey held the office of Lord Mayor in 1577–78. Sir Wolstan Dixie was Lord Mayor in 1585–86 and was knighted on 6 February 1586.[32] Sir Richard Martin's service as Lord Mayor was unusual in that he served two partial terms. His first term came in 1589, when he was called to complete the term of Sir Martin Calthorpe, who had died on 5 May 1589. His second tenure of office came on the first of July, 1594, upon the death of Sir Cuthbert Buckle.[33]

With the possible exception of Ramsey, all the presidents also served as either wardens or masters of their respective guilds. The guilds were very powerful in sixteenth-century London and their leadership provided important experience for future City officials.

> By far the greatest influence which the companies possessed was the control which they exercised over the citizenship of the metropolis. . . . The great body of citizens of London, however, became such through their membership in a company. This was effected in three ways. The person might be made free by serving as an apprentice, or by showing that he was the son of a freeman of London, or by receiving the privilege through purchase or by gift.[34]

Offley became master of the Merchant Taylors from 1547 to 1548.[35] Dixie was a member of the Skinner's Company and was the master of that company in 1573, 1576, 1580, 1583, 1586, 1588, and 1592.[36] Martin was a goldsmith and was the prime warden of his company in 1592–93.[37]

The majority of the presidents of Christ's Hospital were not native Londoners. "[L]ess than one in ten of the greater merchants is known to have been born in London, and three-quarters of the Elizabethan mayors were first-generation Londoners."[38] This is a significant fact, because it demonstrates that Tudor London's political and social structure was fluid and not rigidly controlled by a few powerful families. Sixteenth-century London was a place where new men and new ideas could find a home. Among the presidents of Christ's, Offley "was eldest son of William Offley, a native of Staffordshire, who afterward migrated to Chester, and became sheriff there in 1517."[39] Dixie was the fourth son of "Thomas Dixie and Anne Jephson of Catworth in Huntingdonshire, born in 1525. His ancestors had been seated at Catworth for several generations. . . ."[40] As evidenced by the presidents of Christ Hospital, it was not at all unusual for a young man from the provinces to migrate to London and to become successful and powerful. There was no such thing as great merchant family dynasties during the Tudor century.

> The aldermanic families of London in the 1550s and 1560s bore names unfamiliar at the Guildhall a generation earlier and hardly known there in the fifteenth century. In fact, of the lord mayors in the 55 years 1530–85, only ten were sons of freemen of London. . . The fluidity of the merchant class, already marked in the fifteenth century, was thus no less pronounced in the sixteenth.[41]

The presidents of Christ's Hospital also discharged a variety of positions for the other hospitals. In addition to his work at Christ's as governor starting in 1573–74, Dixie was an auditor and governor of Bridewell for one year in 1576–77 and was president of Bridewell in 1589.[42] Sir Wolstan Dixie was also surveyor general of the hospitals in 1592–94. Marten's service to the hospitals prior to his election as president consisted of sporadic governorships of Christ's and Bridewell. He was also comptroller general of the hospitals from 1594–1602.

Having assessed the various public positions held by the presidents of Christ's Hospital, let me try to describe more fully their careers and their position in London society.

Sir Thomas Offley was president from 1559 to 1563. He was born in Stafford, probably in 1505, and died on 29 August 1582. At the age of twelve Offley went to London, where he studied under William Lily of Jesus School in Paul's Church Yard. "He was apprenticed at an early age to a merchant tailor and merchant of the staple, named John Mechels, described as an intimate friend of Lily."[43] Offley also served as a governor of Bridewell from 1564–65 until 1560–1570, and was comptroller general of the hospitals from 1570-71 until 1575-76. On 7 February 1556/57 he was knighted. He was married once, to Joan Nichells or Nichols, perhaps the daughter of the John Mechels, under whom he served his apprenticeship. Only one son, Henry, survived him. Offley was renowned for his generosity to various charities.[44] According to Stow, he "appointed by his testament the one half of all his goods, and two hundred pounds deducted out of the other half given to his son Henry, to be given and bestowed in deeds of charity by his executors, according to his confidence and trust in them."[45] In 1582, probably as a bequest of this will, £100 was given to Christ's Hospital in his name.[46]

Sir Thomas Ramsey was the president of Christ's Hospital from 1582–83 until his death on 19 May 1590. Ramsey was a member of the Grocer's Guild. Sir Thomas's service to the hospitals was not limited to Christ's; he was also governor and auditor for St. Barts from 1559–60 until 1560–61 and in 1578–79 and 1581–82. Before his term as president of Christ's, Ramsey had served as a governor of St. Bartholomew's from 1559–60 until 1560–61. He also served as an auditor for St. Barts in 1560–61. Ramsey was surveyor general from 1586 until 1590.[47] "His widow (daughter of William Dale, of Bristol), was a benefactress to Christ's Hospital and to Queen Elizabeth's Hospital, Bristol."[48] Ramsey left £20 in his will to Christ's.[49]

Sir Wolstan Dixie was elected president of Christ's Hospital in 1590 and filled that office until his death on 8 January 1594.[50] "He appears to have been apprenticed to Sir Christopher Draper of the Ironmongers' Company."[51] He married a daughter of his ex-master, who was a former Lord Mayor and governor of St. Thomas Hospital.[52] He left many charitable legacies in his will; they illustrate not only his generosity but his many interests as well:

> a fund for establishing a divinity lecture at the church of St. Michael Bassishaw, in which parish he resided; 500Li. to the Skinners' Company to lend at a low rate of interest to young merchants; money for coals to the poor of his parish; annuities to St. Bartholomew's and St. Thomas's Hospitals; money for the poor in Bridewell, Newgate, and the prison in Southwark; for the two compters, and to Ludgate and Bedlam; 100Li. to portion four maids; 50Li. to the strangers of the French and Dutch churches; 200Li. towards building a pesthouse; besides provision for the poor of his parish and of Ealing, where he had a house, on the day of his funeral.[53]

At a governors' meeting on 15 January 1593/94 necessitated by the death of Dixie, a new president was chosen: at "ye said place ye right worshipful Sir Richard Martin knight ye chiefest" was named "governour of this house."[54] Martin was president of Christ's Hospital from 1594 until 1602, when he was succeeded by Sir Stephen Slaney.[55] Sir Richard Martin was born in 1534 and died in 1617. "In 1559-60 he was appointed warden of the mint, and held this office till 1594-5, and perhaps later. In 1580–81 he was appointed master of the mint, and appears to have held this office till his death in 1617."[56] Being master of the mint was not an unmixed monetary blessing, and the holding of that office apparently was the cause of his removal from his aldermanship in 1602. "[T]he reasons assigned [were] his poverty and imprisonment for debt, and his refusal to surrender his office after having accepted one thousand marks as a condition of his retirement."[57] Eight years later Martin was still correcting his affairs. "On 11 Sept. 1610 Martin received a warrant from James I for the repayment of £410 still due to him as warden of the mint under Elizabeth."[58]

The presidents of all the hospitals in general, and Christ's in particular, were distinguished men with vast experience within the Corporation, in Parliament, within their guilds, within their parishes, and in all aspects of life in their city. One would be hard-pressed to name men of the time with more distinguished personal and professional credentials than the eight men who served as the presidents of Christ's during the period of this study. Their stature reflects that of the hospital itself.

The treasurers of Christ's Hospital during the course of the years covered by this book were Richard Grafton, printer (1552–57); Richard Buckland, clothworker (1557–59); Robert Cage, salter (1559–61); John Jackson (1561–73); William Leonard, mercer (1573); Thomas Hall, salter (1573–1582); William Norton, stationer (1582–93); and Robert Cogan, clothworker (1593–1614).[59]

> Each hospital also had a treasurer, who was always a common councilman. Should a councilman gain election to the Court of Alderman while treasurer, he resigned the latter in favour of another councilman. Among the four auditors-general of the hospitals, after the mid-1560s two were aldermen and two councilmen. Their broad supervisory authority extended to all hospitals; there was no attempt to associate each auditor-general with one of the hospitals.[60]

It is difficult to gauge adequately the careers and accomplishments of the treasurers, with the exception of Richard Grafton. They were not as prominent as the presidents or some of the other governors. Beaven doesn't give information on them, because they were not aldermen, and the *Dictionary of National Biography* does not list them, because they were not notable. The hospital needed men who could serve as treasurer for long periods of time and whose energies would not be dissipated by other concerns, such as running a City ward or providing leadership for a guild.

Richard Grafton officiated as the hospital's first treasurer from 1552 to 1555 and was the most prominent man to hold that office. He was a member of Parliament three times, sitting for London in 1553–54 and 1556–57 and once for Coventry in 1562–63. Grafton was best known as a printer, although he was also a merchant and a grocer, serving as warden of that company in 1555 and 1556.[61]

> In November 1538 Coverdale's corrected English translation of the New Testament, with the Latin text, was "printed in Paris by Francis Regnault . . . for Richard Grafton and Edward Whitchurch, citizens of London." . . . This is the earliest book bearing Grafton's name. But Grafton and Whitchurch chiefly concentrated their attention on the folio Bible, known as "the Great Bible." . . .[62]

Richard Grafton had a printing press in the confines of the Greyfriars Monastery, where he printed *The Primer* in 1540. Grafton would continue operating a printing press after Greyfriars became Christ's Hospital in 1552.[63] In fact, Grafton paid an annual rent of £6 13s. 4d. "for his printing house for one whole year ended at Michaelmas in anno 1562."[64] He printed an impressive list of books after the publication of *The Great Bible:* "the first book of Homilies in 1547, the first Book of Common Prayer in 1549, and the edition of 1552, and 'Acts of Parliament' in 1552 and 1553."[65] Grafton is also known for his *Chronicle at large and mere History of the Affairs of England,* which was first published in 1568.[66] In addition to serving as treasurer to Christ's Hospital, Grafton was surveyor of land belonging to Christ's (1558, 1561–62) and overseer of ordinary collection (1560). He was also a governor of Bridewell from 1559 to 1561. Grafton seems to have experienced economic difficulties; for reasons that are unclear, he couldn't pay the rent for his printing house in 1565–66 and again in 1568.[67] Grafton and the hospital had a dispute over a piece of land that required the intervention of the Court of Aldermen in December of 1571 and May of 1572.

> [I]t was agreed that Mr Jackson one of the governors of Christ's Hospital shall make an entry in & upon that piece of void ground at the Greyfriars which Richard Grafton of long time hath wrongfully kept from the poor that upon the same ground there may be built a house wherein the sick persons of Christ's Hospital may be kept from the whole.[68]

This settlement may have taken place after Grafton's death, for he died sometime in 1572.[69]

Richard Buckland, in addition to serving as treasurer of Christ's, functioned as the treasurer of Bridewell from 1566–67 until 1571–72. Before becoming treasurer of Christ's, Buckland was its undertreasurer in 1556–57. Foster, in his *Politics of Stability: A Portrait of the Rulers in Elizabethan London,* lists him as a haberdasher. He served on the common council from 1558 to 1571.[70]

There is some confusion about the identity of Mr. Cage. Both the Book of Legacies and Pearce list a Robert Cage, salter, as treasurer from 1559 to 1561. However, the Minutes of the Court of Governors records the selection of one Anthony Cage as treasurer for the fiscal year of 1559–60.[71]

John Jackson was treasurer of the hospital during the twelve years between 1561/62 and 1572/73. He also served as one of eight "Surveyors of all the lands and tenements belonging to Christ's Hospital" in 1561–62.[72]

A mercer named William Leonard was elected as treasurer on 21 September 1573 for the upcoming fiscal year. A month later, however, a new treasurer was needed due to the death of Leonard. Thomas Hall was elected the new treasurer of Christ's Hospital on 30 October 1573. It was the death of Leonard and the troublesome process of finding a new treasurer that prompted the governors to reassert that no one should serve the hospital as treasurer "except they [were] willing to serve the full of 2 years according to a former order in that behalf."[73]

Thomas Hall was a good choice as the new treasurer. He had experience as a governor and auditor of St. Bartholomew's Hospital from 1566–67 until the date of his election as treasurer, and had just been reelected governor and auditor of St. Barts when he assumed the new position. Hall was treasurer for eight years and served for part of the 1581–82 fiscal year. Sometime during that year William Norton fully assumed his responsibilities, most probably due to Hall's death. The Book of Legacies lists a donation of £4 to Christ's in 1582, in the form of a "house in Breadstreet." This donation was probably a provision of his will.[74]

William Norton was treasurer of the hospital from 1581–82 until 1593, the probable date of his death. The Book of Legacies lists a gift in 1593—"Master William Norton Stationer Houses in Seacoal Lane etc"—without specifying the amount such a donation was worth.[75] However, property given to Christ's by Norton yielded an annual rent of £20 in 1595/96.[76]

Robert Cogan was treasurer of Christ's from 1593–94 until 1614.[77] Prior to his election as treasurer, Cogan served Bridewell as a governor from 1582–83 until 1586–87 and also in 1592–93. Administrative stability was provided by the long-term service of the presidents and treasurers of Christ's.

Among other governors of Christ's who held a variety of offices was Robert Broke, grocer, who, while serving as a governor for Christ's in 1583–

84, and 1586–87, was also a member of Parliament representing the city of York. John Hayden, mercer, was a governor of Christ's from 1577–78 until his death in 1582. Stow records that Hayden "gave large legacies, more than three thousand pounds, for the relief of the poor. . . . "[78]

Most of the governors served for more than one yearly term. This makes sense from a purely practical vantage point. The hospital would need a core of experienced governors whose expertise could be relied upon year after year. Having to introduce to the operations of the orphanage too many new governors each year would have diverted energy more properly spent upon the children. The City, in its recording of the official election results, takes pains to make the distinction between those who are newly elected and "those that continued one year and must remain another," indicating that it was expected that governors would serve at least two years.[79] Howes in his *Contemporaneous Account, in Dialogue Form of the Foundation and Early History of Christ's Hospital and of Bridewell and St. Thomas' Hospitals*, claims that five to seven years was the length of service for governors.

> *Dignity* asks "Then sir I pray you show me what is the reason why the Governors continue 5, 6, or 7 years in one house knowing that there is a constitution & a promise made to the king to avoid the suspicion & occasion of corruption that they shall change & shift their governors every year or two year at ye most."
>
> *Dutie* replies "There hath of late been some occasion offered by reason of a suit which continued long & besides if they should stay but one year they could never enter into the secrets of the government, nor understand ye state of the house & so altogether unable to accomplish that which is looked for at their hands."[80]

It was not unusual for at least two aldermen to sit as governors of Christ's during their term of office. This is a reflection of the time demands upon the governors; it was a seriously regarded "part-time job." Governors could also serve as aldermen while president of the hospital, but it was unusual to serve in any other major City position. There are two exceptions, and they concern residing Lord Mayors who were elected to hospital offices during the term of their mayoralty. The first case is that of Sir Thomas Pullison, who had a long record of service to Christ's starting in 1570–71. He was president of Bridewell from 1586 to 1588, and was a governor of the orphanage during his mayoralty. At the general court meeting to elect hospital officials on 21 September 1585, Thomas Pullison, a draper, was selected as a governor "and yet Lord Mayor," although he still had another week of his mayoralty left until the annual Michaelmas City election.[81] Although the overlap of authority was for a limited time period, it was still a violation of practice and no explanation is given for this departure from normal procedure. The second case is that of Sir Thomas Cambell, ironmonger, who filled the office of sheriff while still governor of the hospital in 1600–1601. Cambell filled the mayoralty of London in 1609–10 and was also a governor of East India Company in 1602–3. Christ's Hospital was not the only school that held the interest of its governors; many were drawn to support other educational endeavors. Sir Wolstan Dixie was not only generous to his other charities, as detailed above, but was interested in supporting schools. "He had subscribed 50 Li. towards the building of the new puritan college of Emmanuel in Cambridge (1584), and in his will he left 600 Li. to purchase land to endow two fellowships and two scholarships for the scholars of his new grammar school at Market Bosworth."[82] Sir Richard Marten became a governor of the Highgate free school in 1562, the year of its foundation by Sir Roger Cholmeley.[83] Thomas Aldersey, an M.P. in the parliaments of 1572 and 1581, and who served as governor of Christ's, Bridewell, and St. Thomas, "in 1593 had constituted a great endowment for the founding of a grammer school in his native town of Burbury, Cheshire. . . . "[84] Sir William Harper, merchant tailor, who filled the offices of sheriff in 1556–57 and Lord Mayor in 1561–62, "helped to found the Merchant Tailors' School, which was established during his mayoralty. . . ."[85] In addition, on 22 April 1566 Harper and his wife, Alice, granted by indenture to the mayor and corporation of his native city of Bedford a piece of land with school buildings upon it. For the support of the school and other charitable objectives she left thirteen acres and one rood of meadow land in the parish of St. Andrew, Holborn.[86] An interest in other foundations of learning was not reserved exclusively to the governors. James Peele, clerk of Christ's from 1563–85, was granted "ye sum of twenty pounds, . . . by order of court in consideration that he desolved his private school which he kept, in his house. . . ."[87] The governors and other men associated with Christ's Hospital felt strongly enough about education to make generous endowments to all types of schools. It is difficult to conclude whether this interest stemmed from immediate personal concerns, represented a feeling of general obligation reflecting their positions as leaders of their community, or embodied a combination of both.

The governors not only donated their time without compensation but could be relied upon to advance money for a loan to the hospital and to remember it in their wills. For example in the 1586–87 fiscal year, twenty-eight governors lent £165 to the hospital "to supply ye great charges thereof, until it shall please God to make this house able to repay ye same again. . . ."[88] Christ's president, Sir Thomas Ramsey, Sir Wolstan Dixie, Alderman Martin Calthrop, Alderman Stephen Slany, and Alderman Henry Pranell each contributed £10. Richard Gourney, Henry Isham, Baldwin Derham, James Hewishe, Robert Brooke, Richard Bowdler, Thomas Laurence, Thomas Ware, Thomas Audley, Mr. Gawdbie, Thomas Tomlinson, John Highlorde, Robert Hawes, Oliver Rowe, Thomas Alderseie, Roger Clercke, Thomas Cambell, Humphrey Huntley, John Blounte, John Southall, John Burnell, Thomas Banks, and John Stoyer each gave £5. Sometimes, the lending governors did not require repayment. Such was the case with the loan of Thomas Aldersey, a wealthy haberdasher. "At this court master Aldersey one of the governors of this house who hereto foreseeing the want of Christ's Hospital did lend to master treasurer to the relief of the children the sum of £L which £L he doth at this court absolutely give to this house."[89]

The hospitals provided a two-pronged opportunity for their governors: to do good deeds by helping the poor, and to provide status positions for the London elite. The presidency of the hospitals and the governorships allowed men with vast experience to exercise their talents beyond the confines of their trades and daily lives and to serve their fellow Londoners in a useful, productive, and visible capacity. Although the governors of Christ's and the other hospitals were drawn from a small elite, their charges came from a variety of backgrounds and circumstances. These same men who served as governors of the royal hospitals not only gave money to the cause but gave their time, energy, and, above, all a guiding sense of purpose.

6

The Children

> It is the ancient Greyfriars' Church, which the king my father hath taken from the monks and given for a home forever for poor and forsaken children. . . .

This synopsis of the background and purpose of Christ's Hospital was uttered by Edward Tudor, the founder of the orphanage, in Mark Twain's, *The Prince and the Pauper*. However, a great deal more needs to be said about these orphans other than to describe them as "poor and forsaken." A number of questions come immediately to mind. What children were eligible? How did they come to fall under the protection of this orphanage? What happened to these children after adolescence? This chapter will focus on the children and will examine these questions and others, although it is a task that often proves frustrating. For example, one cannot even assume that the children in the hospital were orphans, which is, after all, the definition of an orphanage. As with everything else relating to Christ's, simple answers do not present themselves even to simple questions. Christ's Hospital opened its doors to a variety of children in difficult and life-threatening circumstances. This institution tended to the needs of sick, disabled, abandoned, or just plain poor children, whether orphaned or not. Some of these children were the sons and daughters of married London citizens, some were foundlings, some were the children of unwed mothers or criminals. Some were infants, toddlers, or even adolescents. Some required only temporary assistance. Some of the children didn't even reside within the walls of the hospital. However, two broad categorizations can be made: children were admitted to Christ's Hospital either because their own condition placed them in immediate peril or because of parental exigency.

The information provided in this chapter is taken from the Children's Register, which contains a portrait of these children's lives.[1] The information there is anecdotal and offers a unique insight into the lives of ordinary children, a group of people not usually represented in historical records. A typical entry in the Children's Register contains such facts as the name of the child; the father's name and occupation; the age of the child; the parish or individual who requested admission; whether the child was kept in residence or sent to nurse; and if the child was put to service, adopted, returned to parents, or died. These excellent records were kept so that the governors could quickly locate a child when needed, and have the essential information at hand when decisions were made concerning the child. Once again, it needs to be stressed that the orphanage was not intended to be a place where unwanted children could be handed over to indifferent caregivers to be neglected and forgotten. The hospital kept track of these children because it mattered to the City what happened to them in their battle against poverty and vagrancy. Christ's was the place "where the poor children [were] trained in the knowledge of God and some virtuous exercise, to the overthrow of beggary."[2]

The orphanage was originally designed to care for the fatherless children who had been born in London and were at least four years old. However, the need was so great that foundlings and children of all ages who were not born in London were also rescued. The formal statement of the admission requirements suggests a rigidity that did not exist in attitude nor application:

> that ye admit none but such as shall first bring you a bill declaring the child to be above the age of 4 years, and to be born within the city of London, and the child of a free man being destitute of all friends and parents and in danger of present perishing and the same to be subscribed with the hand of 6 of the honestest and substantialest persons of that parish from whence that child cometh and the hand of the alderman. . . .[3]

The governors were not supposed to let the number of children surpass 150 infants and 250 older children. It is not clear if that is the in-house population or the total. This was the ideal as formulated in 1556, but seems to have been honored more in its breach; by the end of the century, the hospital had assumed the responsibility for over six hundred children.[4] "In the 1580s and 1590s Christ's catered for between 550 and 650 children at any one time, representing an annual intake of between 60 and 90."[5] It is to the credit of the governors that a direct personal appeal would often result in admittance, even if the orphanage was at its full capacity. After all, the governors were not made of stone and a touching story was probably as effective then as now. In other words, the governance of Christ's Hospital was not so bureaucratized that room could not be found for one more.

In addition to the governors themselves, local officials could circumvent normal procedure and successfully petition admission for children. The Lord Mayor, the Court of Aldermen, and the bishop of London were able to order the admittance of children *ex officio.*

> Although the children of freemen were clearly preferred, its admissions policy was reasonably broad . . . the frequently expressed reluctance to admit illegitimates was regularly overcome as foundlings accounted for about 10 per cent of those admitted by the end of the century. The majority of the children, sponsored by the parish vestries, came from one-parent families of households overburdened with children.[6]

Having dealt with the administrative apparatus, we can now turn to the children whose health or predicament placed them in danger. Those perceived at risk were the youngsters who were sick, disabled, abandoned, or engaged in criminal behavior.

Suffering from a host of illnesses, sick children were routinely admitted and given treatment "where loss of life and perishing would presently follow, if they [were] not received into this said hospital. . . ."[7] From the beginning, Christ's had medical expertise; the first surgeon appointed "was Robert Ballthorp who became sergeant surgeon to Queen Elizabeth. . . ."[8] The orphanage did possess on-site medical facilities in the form of a sick ward supervised by the matron and nurses, with physicians and surgeons available when needed. For example, on 7 April 1593, in the aftermath of an especially virulent outbreak of the plague, the governors agreed to grant to surgeon William Martine a benevolence of forty shillings "in consideration of his great charges expended in surgery upon the sick. . . ."[9]

The following examples are randomly selected to give a general idea of the illnesses that were deemed serious enough for admission. Richard Robynson, age not given, was "taken up in the streets being swollen very sore in the body in consideration of his extremity" and admitted.[10] On 14 April 1576, sixteen-year-old Elizabeth Watson, described as a "sometime child of this House . . . and having the bloody flux and wanting succor" was admitted."[11] An epileptic child was admitted: "Dick Fool, a woman child of 12 years or there about being a very innocent having the falling sickness and taken up in the streets."[12] (The name or the gender is mistakenly identified here.) Starvation or its threat was also considered as a medical emergency requiring immediate attention. Thus the records refer to "a woman child starving which was taken at Billingsgate from a poor woman and sent in by Sir William Chester knight."[13]

As might be expected from the discussion of the deserving poor in the introduction, disabled children, especially those blind and lame, received exceptional consideration. Robert Goodmanne, a twenty-year-old blind youth who had been under the care of Christ's since he was four, was successfully apprenticed "to Richard Wilson Clerk of this Hospital, 8 years, and by him put over to William Smith minstrel of Claiton Well and to him was paid in money towards his education 40s."[14] Disabled children were not necessarily admitted to the hospital itself but were given aid and permitted to reside with a parent. "Sometimes Christ's actually put the children out to nurse to their own parents, providing a form of family allowance and access to the hospital facilities."[15] Such was the case with John Hickoxe: "a child of this house being fallen lame is by consent of this court [sent] unto his mother Elizabeth Hickoxe until he be recovered . . . and she to have 8d. weekly for the keeping of him."[16]

Another special category of children admitted into the hospital were foundlings. The admission of abandoned infants posed a difficult dilemma for hospital authorities: they could hardly let these babies die, yet by accepting responsibility for foundlings, they unintentionally encouraged desperate mothers to abandon children in the expectation that Christ's would take care of them. Thus a vicious cycle ensued whereby the more foundlings were rescued, the more foundlings were literally dropped on the doorstep. The admission of foundlings also extraordinarily taxed the limited resources of the hospital because, as it was unlikely that a parent or relative would come forward and reclaim an abandoned child. This left Christ's to raise the child until maturity and thereby committed the institution more thoroughly than the relieving of the children of widows; such children might only need temporary support until their mothers remarried. It may have also been that for civic leaders foundlings were not an abstract problem but a situation that confronted them directly in the form of a child left on or near their houses—a not infrequent occurrence, for children were rarely deserted at Christ's itself but all over all the City. Leaving a child on the doorstep of a prominent citizen proved to be an effective tactic for procuring entrance to Christ's. For example, Edward Hewis, gentleman, agreed to donate to Christ's four pence monthly for a period of two years toward the care of an infant found near his house "and thereupon requested that it should be named Katherine Fortune for that it was taken up upon St.

Katherines day at night. . . ."[17] Of course, it could be argued that these men were targeted because they were the fathers; however, this is unlikely and there is no documentation to support that assumption. However, when all is said and done, foundlings elicited special concern, as well they should have, since they were in immediate peril of dying after having been exposed for indeterminate periods of time.

The records permit easy identification of abandoned babies. The names given them usually reflected the place where they were discovered. One-year-old Benedick Fenchurch was so named because he was sent from the parish of Fenchurch and "was laid at Mr. Benedick's gate. . . ."[18] As we have seen with Katherine Fortune, the foundlings' names sometimes indicated the day they were discovered. This was also the case with Valentine Woodyarde: "a young infant very weak being laid at the woodyard door of this House of the age of 5 or 6 weeks old upon St. Valentine's Day in the morning last past. . . ."[19]

The optimal situation, albeit completely unrealistic, would be the evidential identification of at least one biological parent of all abandoned children. There were a few cases where that did occur. The father of John Watson, aged one month, abandoned "in the parish of St. Albans in Wood Street,"[20] turned out to be a smith named Peacock living in the parish of St. Giles. From the vantage point of the hospital administration, a satisfactory arrangement was reached when John's father submitted a bond providing for his son's expenses. Even more unusual, both parents of Anne Orphant Honnings, a three-month-old child found at the gate of Mr. Honnings, were located "by confession of the mother the strumpet Julian Randole. This child's father [was] servant with John Smith butcher in St. Nicholas Shambles. . . ."[21]

Sometimes, foundlings were left with distinctive clothing or a note, the contents of which would be recorded in the register; the parental motivation would appear to be that unique identification would make future reclamation easier. But rather than serving as a realistic strategy for the reunification of their family, this might have simply been a gesture to relieve guilt by mimicking the story of Moses. Such was the case with Moses Dodd, "a very young infant which was laid at the door of Mr. Dodd in St. Albans parish in Wood Street wrapped in a piece of linen and the fore part of a red petticoat and a piece of a shirt and a double cloth on the head of it. . . ."[22] Sometimes, the parent gave the child a name. Such was the case with Susan Cloyster "a young infant of a year and a half or there about, who was yesterday . . . evening left in the westside of the cloister in her bosom a piece of old parchment wherein her name written. . . . "[23]

Children did not have to be babies in order to be abandoned; forsaken older children could also find themselves under the care of Christ's. Thus there is mention of a four-year-old boy named "Robert Pouell whose father and mother [had] run a way a bill found in his bosom being left. . . ."[24] William Fryse, aged twelve, must have also been abandoned; he was brought to the hospital by a sheriff after he was "taken out of the streets begging. . . ."[25]

Older children seem to have posed problems for the hospital. Some of them had difficulty reconciling themselves to their new situation and ran away. John Sympson, who had been under the care of the hospital since he was twelve, ran away when he was fifteen and was not heard from again.[26] Valentine Haines was fifteen years old when he ran away from the orphanage, where he had lived since the age of eighteen months. The last entry for him is "1578 March 29, Home. Ran away."[27] William Skelton ran away when he was seventeen; he had been fifteen when "taken now up in the streets and admitted."[28] It was the policy of Christ's to accept runaways back into its fold when caught, as was the case with "George Lewes, a great boy which ran from this House [who] was sent from Bridewell by the Governors there and admitted."[29] The governors' concern over disappearing children was not a penchant for orderly bookkeeping, but rather their belief that their responsibility to the children was not discharged until the children reached the age of maturity. They did not dismiss their charges at the first available chance and then forget about them, but had a continuing concern, even after the children had left the hospital for training or further schooling. Thus with Richard Howchen aged twelve, "taken out of the streets," we are told: "This child was again delivered to David Couper leatherseller in Tormell Street who is his master, the 24th May 1560."[30] Besides, having their charges flee from their care defeated one of the purposes of the institution: that of keeping parentless children off the streets, where they would become criminals or beggars.

Not all of the older children could be reformed after spending time on the streets. Fourteen-year-old Marie Allin, for instance, ran away from her master on the same day she was placed under his care on a trial basis. Presumably this was the first time she had tried to escape, for she had only been assigned to Christ's the year before, after having been "taken out of the streets abegging."[31] Another incorrigible child was William Lee, who had been with the hospital since the age of ten. When he reached eighteen, he was apprenticed for eight years to a stationer named Robert Lewis, who brought back William two years later because "he ran so often away, and sent to the lime work at Bridewell."[32]

It was not necessarily the condition of the children themselves but parental misfortune encompassing circumstances other than the death of a father that could result in admission to the hospital. Having parents who were either sick or disabled or abandoned left a child as a *de facto* orphan. Therefore, if we define an orphan as one whose parents are not able to properly take care of him/her, then the hospital's policies make more sense. The illness of a parent was a not uncommon predicament that could place children at risk. It acted as guardian if the parent was in the care of one of the other City hospitals. The following infant was admitted because his mother was confined to the City madhouse: "Robert Bethelem, 12 days, son of a mad woman delivered of him in Bedlem."[33] Children whose mothers died while in one of the City hospitals were placed in the care of the orphanage. "Margaret, 1, whose mother died in St. Thomas Hospital taken out of the streets and by them sent in."[34] Two-year-old George Kemberley entered Christ's because he was "the child of a poor and sick woman who died in St. Bartholomews. . . ."[35]

Although each of the City hospitals was run independently, the inter-institutional cooperation is indicated by the fact that Christ's Hospital accepted the children of mothers incarcerated in the various City prisons. Elizabeth Norton, one-and-a-half years old, became a child of the hospital as she was the daughter "of a woman in the Counter prisoner. . . ."[36] Offspring of women who had died in prison were also admitted: "Marko Smymkins, 8 weeks, daughter of a poor woman who died in childbed in Newgate, admitted from the Lord Mayor Mr. George Barnes mayor."[37]

The City even took responsibility for children orphaned as a result of the exercise of the legal apparatus of the City. Isabel Peter, aged thirteen, and Alice Peter, aged eleven, were admitted at the order of the Lord Mayor because their mother was "an Egyptian [gypsy] executed at Tyburn."[38] To the modern reader it may seem like a contradiction to kill the mother but take care of the children, but it wasn't to the government of London. Gypsies were persecuted in England, as they were elsewhere in Europe, because they were perceived as a danger to the social order. By executing the mother of these children, the authorities were ridding themselves of a person who was, by definition, a thief, beggar, and heretic. However, the girls (they thought) could be redeemed and admission to the orphanage prevented them from following in their mother's unorthodox activities.

Not only widows, but also women whose husbands had deserted them, could apply for assistance for their children from Christ's. Loss of a husband either through death or desertion placed the woman in the category of impotent poor. On 14 October 1564, two-year-old Humphrey Adlington, entered the hospital as one "whose father is run away. . . ."[39]

There were a myriad of circumstances that could overwhelm familial resources, and one such situation was simply having too many children. Nine-year-old Dorothy Brooker came back to Christ's on 23 February 1571/72 "for that the mother is frantic and hath six children more and not able to keep them. . . ."[40] Robert and Edward Daie, three-week-old twins whose father was deceased, were put to wet nurse to Jane Mace of Bishopsgate one month after coming under the care of Christ's in 1582. Mrs. Daie, apparently to recover from childbirth, went to stay with friends.[41]

Some children were admitted as a result of parental irresponsibility rather than misfortune. If the parents were engaged in activities that were frowned upon, especially prostitution and beggary, they could have their children taken from them and placed in the hospital, while they themselves would be punished. This was perceived as a preventative measure to save children from following their parents into criminal careers. For example, "Elizabeth Thurstone alias Gryffin, 14, and Christian Tauerner, 8, taken from Alice Gryffin in Turnagain Lane a beggar which Christian brought unto her by begging within 5 days, 22d. and for keeping these to begging she was sent unto Bridewell."[42]

Employees of the orphanage and other hospitals could claim services for their own children. The admission of employee's children may have been an example of the hospital taking care of its own as a sort of fringe benefit or it may demonstrate employees' knowledge of how the system worked and how to manipulate the admissions policy to their advantage. Jane Huggens, aged three, was admitted into the hospital on 11 April 1573 because her mother, Alice, was "one of the nurses of this House. . . ."[43] John Atkinson, aged eight, the son of Maryann, a Christ's Hospital's nurse, was conditionally admitted on 27 May 1581 "upon his mothers diligent service to continue. . . ."[44] Nine-year-old Richard Watson came into Christ's on 1 June 1565 because his father, John was "sometime Clerk of this Hospital. . . ."[45] Employees of the other hospitals could also gain their children's admittance, as was the case with Martin Throgmerton's three-year-old-daughter, Jane, who became a child of Christ's on 3 June 1570 because he was the clerk of Bridewell.[46]

The children of soldiers could command care from the orphanage. Discharged soldiers were traditionally left to fend for themselves after their employer no longer required an army. These soldiers frequently had to find their way back home from foreign lands, without having been paid, leaving them to beg, borrow, or steal their way back. Once home, it was often difficult for them to resume their former lives. "Even those who were officially discharged found it hard to find employment on coming home, and frequently ended up as vagabonds."[47] Under the Statute of Henry VIII in 1531, soldiers were among those deemed worthy to be granted licenses making it legal for them to beg.[48] This established a precedent for regarding ex-soldiers as impotent poor and worthy of some kind of assistance. Queen Elizabeth I ordered the admission of Anthony Wood, five years old, who was the son of "Wood slain in Her Majesties affairs. . . ." [49] Oliver Knolls "late a soldier at Guynes," was given a pension of eight pence weekly for his two children in 1558.[50] Fauarias Bell, aged 7, became a child of Christ's Hospital on 5 September 1588, in the aftermath of the defeat of the Spanish Armada. The Lord Mayor and the Court of Alderman ordered the admission, remarking that his father, Thomas, was "lately slain in Her Majesties service in the Low Countries. . . ."[51]

Children born in Calais, the last remnant of the Angevin empire in France that had been lost in 1558, elicited special patriotic attention on the part of the governors. Five-year-old Adrian Norrice became a child of Christ's on 15 July 1560; he was "born at Calais and sent in by Mr. Grafton with whom was given 10s."[52] One of the success stories is that of Thomas Colfe, aged seven, "born at Calais taken up in the street and sent in to this House by the Lord Mayor for the time being. . . ." Fifteen years later, in 1578, he was "preferred to Oxford by the Salters Company. . . ."[53]

From time to time, conditions were imposed upon parents in exchange for acceptance of their children. On 12 November 1567, Richard Rodes was placed under the care of the orphanage "until the mother marry." This boy was never reunited with his mother; he died at nurse on 17 July 17 1568 while under the care of Margery Woodfyne.[54] Henry Rotcheford arranged for the admission of Henry Broke, "a starveling of 1 1/2" by promising "2s. a month while the child liveth. . . ." This child died on 21 February 1573/74.[55] "Brian Maperley about the age of vii year being lame on one leg was admitted for surgery at the suit of Richard Cappe his wife a plasterer at Broken Wharf who hath promised to receive him again after that he is recovered."[56]

Hospital authorities would cooperate with citizens to place children, even trading an older child for a younger, especially if that led to an adoption.

> And there is also granted unto John Sowell furrier dwelling in St. Sepulchres parish who had a woman child about the age of one quarter left on his stall that for the admission thereof he should unburden this

House of another named Mathew Thomson of the age of 8 years whom he hath taken for his own.[57]

Once their children were admitted to the guardianship of the orphanage, parents were not required to abandon parental rights nor was future reclamation difficult. Those administering Christ's exercised considerable latitude in carrying out their commitments. In particular, they recognized that parents' inability to support their children might be the result of short-term misfortunes rather than a permanent condition. Thus, children were routinely returned to parents when the situation warranted. In fact, reading the records of admission gives the impression of a revolving door, with children entering and exiting Christ's several times. James Bowle, aged seven at the time of his admission on 13 February 1573/74, resided in Christ's for four years until released "to his parents again and they have discharged the House of him from henceforth."[58]

Although it was not common for other family members to tend to their needy kin, there were a few cases in which uncles would assume responsibility for their nieces and nephews. For example, a goldsmith named Mr. Clerk cared for his nephew, promising "to apparel and put to service a boy named Richard Lybias his sisters son of the age of 12 years taken out of the streets."[59] Eleven-year-old Grace Maior, who had been resident in the hospital since she was one-and-a half, was discharged in 1581 "to her uncle William Maior tailor of St. Peters Cornhill."[60] There was no attempt to force families to care for youngsters other than their own children; extended kin were not expected to automatically become guardians of orphaned relatives.

Some of the children found permanent homes with foster parents. Thomas Farnam, seventeen, was adopted on 15 March 1571/72 by "Thomas Danyell of East Ham fisherman who hath taken him for his own child and discharged this House of him."[61] A ten-year-old boy named John Peacock found a foster mother in Margery Graundger after a false start: "1563 April 13, to Margery Graundger of Hammersmith. April 17, Home. June 12, to Margery Graundger aforesaid with 10s. in ready money and she hath discharged this House of him for ever."[62] Margaret Cottingham, "born in the sheepcote in Smithfield," was six months old when admitted to Christ's. Seven years later, this child was "with Blanche Williamson. 1570 Easter, to the same Blanche Williamson for ever."[63]

There did not seem to be a stringent rule, but somewhere in adolescence, the children were either put to service or apprenticed. That was the second step in Christ's charge. Having been placed within the care of

Christ's, the children received a basic education designed to provide them with the essentials for learning a trade when of age. "A degree of functional literacy was expected of apprentices in many companies, especially those associated with the city's retail, wholesale, and overseas trades, since an apprentice often ran the shop in his master's absence."[64] The salters' company issued an order in 1581 that "no man being in the clothing or out of the clothing shall take new apprentices without he can write and read. . . ."[65] In addition, the children had instruction in music and religion.

Youngsters put to service entered a casual and less complicated relationship than apprenticeship. For example, William Semar was seventeen when he entered into the following arrangement on 20 June 1579:

> to Robert Browne barber surgeon, 9 yrs. Put over from Mr. Browne to one Braswell an instrument maker of St. Clements without Temple Bar for 9 years aforesaid and it is agreed that Semar shall become covenanted servant with the said Braswell for meat drink and clothing and £4 the year.[66]

Apprenticeship required a formal contractual arrangement between the child, the master, and the hospital. Apprenticeship agreements were legally binding and were contracted for the protection of both the adult and the child. They specified length of service and any special conditions, which was standard practice by the guilds and also demonstrates the thoroughness with which the governors exercised their protective duty. "In the 1580s an average of thirty-three children a year left the hospital for apprenticeship or service, sometimes in the household of prominent citizens."[67]

> The treasurer, with one other of the governors at the least, shall put forth any of the children of this house to service, having a careful regard to whom they be put; chiefly, that they be honest persons, and such as be well able to keep them, and to bring them up to such faculty, service or occupation, as they may hereafter be good members in the commonwealth . . . and that as nigh as they can, to bind them with none, but with freemen of this city; and before they be so put forth, being men children, they may write and read and cast accounts. . . .[68]

John Moore, fourteen, was first apprenticed on 8 October 1598 "to James Bull buttonmaker and Alice his wife, 8 years." The record comments, "Put this child to John Fasty to be his prentice for 10 years to serve him as a mariner and to be bound in the Admiralty: his dwelling is at Barking in Essex."[69]

The boys of Christ's entered into service arrangements in the same manner as any other young men, except that they were apprenticed at the earlier age of twelve to sixteen. Steve Rappaport states that

> Most men in London did not begin apprenticeships until they were nearly twenty years old . . . since he earned his own keep while serving his term, an orphan was no longer dependent upon others once he began his training. For orphans, therefore, the pressure to begin apprenticeships early in life might have been considerable.[70]

In addition to beginning at earlier ages, Christ's Hospital children seem to have had a slightly longer term of service; they contracted for seven to ten years, with eight or nine years seeming the most common. This is not far off from Rappaport's findings in his study of apprentices in Tudor London; he concluded that the average length of service was 7.7 years in the minor companies and 8.2 for the great companies.[71]

Although the children were mostly apprenticed to London citizens, some were sent outside the City and were settled in proximate counties such as Middlesex, Essex, Hertford, Buckinghamshire, Surrey, and Suffolk. They were also put out to areas in close proximity to the City: Southwark, St. Giles in the Fields, Smithfield, and Bethnal Green. The cities of Norwich, Ipswich, and Yarmouth became homes for some of the children. The following agreement details a contract for a child placed outside London, nowhere explaining why this child was not placed in a similar situation within the City:

> Melcher Sampton one of the poor children of this Hospital delivered to one John Whitlock of Uxbridge musician to dwell with him for 8 years and he to have at the end of his years of his said master 20s. In ready money and an instrument, for the performance whereof the same John Whitlock and John Edling musicians of Uxbridge with Nicholas Browne merchant tailor stand all bound by obligation to the Governors of this House as by the said bond doth and may appear.[72]

Children were put out to work in a surprisingly diverse range of occupations. Some of these livelihoods included common trades such as embroiderer, barber surgeon, bricklayer, white baker, and carpenter. However, some of Christ's Hospital alumni found careers in professions that sound quaint to modern ears but did necessary work: gunmaker, armorer, compass maker, felt-maker, needlemaker, and bucket maker.[73] There may have been an attempt made to match the child's interests and talent with his or her future trade.

Some of the staff of Christ's Hospital took on apprentices. John Harris was sixteen when on 12 March 1575 he was apprenticed "to Ralph Waddington grammar master in this house and free of the fishmongers for 9 years from the Annunciation of Our Lady 1575."[74] John Jackson was treasurer of Christ's when on 15 September 1571 he arranged to "take an apprentice Elizabeth Trashe a child of this house for from Michaelmas 1571." It was agreed "at Easter next she shall have a new petticoat of the charge of this house."[75] Francis Godlie, aged fifteen, was apprenticed on 8 August 1573 "to Robert Cook, steward of this House, 9 years."[76]

Christ's did not abandon all interest and responsibility when the children's care was transferred to other adults. If an apprenticeship or service arrangement did not work out satisfactorily, the child could come back to the orphanage. The master may have found that an attractive part of the agreement; the master, or for that matter the child, would not be bound to continue a relationship that was not working out. On 21 May 1569, Agnes Sqwier, aged twelve, was put "to service to James Cotts silkweaver of Clerkenwell." On 2 July of the same year, Agnes was readmitted into the hospital "in consideration her master is very sick and the indenture canceled."[77] Eleven-year-old Richard Hartelpoole was apprenticed to John Meris on 6 May 1564. Three years later, this child was returned to the hospital "for that his master is run away."[78] Sometimes the reason for altering service contracts was not recorded. For example, Robert Dent was apprenticed three times. The first apprenticeship, in 1572, was when he was fifteen in 1572. On 27 October 1573, Robert was apprenticed to a haberdasher named Edmund Mathewes. On 7 July 1576, he was "Bound to John Wheler joyner, 7 years."[79] Jane Craiford was at the advanced age of twenty when placed under the care of Christ's; four years later she was put "to service to Nicholas Thornton. This wench is received again from her master."[80] Masters turned over their apprentices to other masters for unspecified reasons on occasion. Hercules Knighte, aged thirteen, was apprenticed on 5 March 1592/93 to Thomas Frier citizen and merchant tailor of London" for a period of ten years "and by him put over to William Smith minstrel, 8 years."[81]

It was hospital policy that when the children's capabilities were judged to warrant it, they received an education preparing them for one of the universities. A few attended Oxford and Cambridge. It should be emphasized that these university students were only a tiny minority of the alumni of Christ's Hospital and the hospital was in no way seen as a preparatory school for the universities. "And that such of the children as be pregnant and very apt to learning, be reserved and kept in the grammar-school, in hope of preferment to University; where they may be virtuously educated. . . ."[82]

While the hospital's reputation was advanced by its academically more able charges and the governors were anxious to encourage and prepare them, attention was also paid to the needs of less able students. A sum of £3 12s was "Paid to George Kinge, and George Pulliard drummers to her Majesty for 3 drums to instruct the ignorant sort of children in which are not apt for their books. . . ."[83] An additional £4 was "Paid to the said drummers for teaching diverse of the children to play one the drum . . . and still continuing in instructing them. . . ."[84]

Although placements were carefully considered and attempts were made to place the children in the best possible circumstance, there were some instances of abuse. A seven-year-old boy named Robert Mills was deliberately injured by his guardian, Mrs. Robert Hill, whose apparent motive was to gain possession of the child's goods: "in whose hands were certain goods left for the child's use as by the bill appeareth which child was by the said woman evil entreated and cast down a pair of stairs and brake his back who was for that offence warned against the next Court."[85] John Hopkings was abused by his master, John Baggett, silkweaver, to whom he was apprenticed since the age of nine. "Received again this child for that he was misgoverned with his master."[86] Isabel Gadd, nine years old, was sent to her father three months after returning to the hospital: "for that she was very ill used, which child was put to service out of this House. . . ."[87] Eramus Hardinge, aged ten, the son of Stephen Hardinge, deceased, returned to the hospital in March of 1566/67 "for that he was very ill used by them that took him. . . ." Although Richard Aston of St. Giles, Cripplegate, adopted him ("hath taken him for his own child"), this child finally found a home with his mother "for good and all."[88] Ellen Parker, aged eight years, was apprenticed on 25 September 1568 "to John Williams baker of Christ Church. Received again from the same John Williams who with unreasonable correction misused her. . . ." Evans Gryffin of Tunbridge then adopted her.[89] Abuse from a fellow child was no more tolerated than if the offense had been perpetrated by an adult. John Pott was ejected from the orphanage itself and was returned to his parents because he "abused one of his wenches in this house"; for this he was "appointed to be punished. . . ."[90]

The records indicate the governors' strong intolerance for any behavior endangering the health or safety of the children. The following situation is a good example of the hospital's quick response when one of their children was in danger:

> Jane St. Thomas . . . 1591 April 24, was put upon liking and within one month after bound . . . to Christopher Moseley and Katherine his wife and continued with them in service until the 16 February 1592, upon which day the said Jane upon information of their neighbours of the grievous and ill usage towards her was by the Matron of Christ's Hospital fetched from them and brought into the nursery of the said Hospital where she died the 24 February 1592 [she was fourteen] . . . the matter is referred to the discretion of the magistrate.[91]

The case of Jane St. Thomas is important for four reasons: first, she was an orphan and probably illegitimate; second, the neighbors complained; third, the governors acted to remove the child from an abusive environment; fourth, after the child's death, the case was referred to other authorities for possible criminal prosecution. The fact that the neighbors complained seems to indicate a general intolerance for the mistreatment of children and hardly supports the theory that children were routinely abused and maltreated.

The governors exercised a great deal of flexibility when deciding the admission, care, and the futures of their charges. They defined the parameters of care rather broadly and went beyond simply caring for destitute children. Their goal was never just to tend physically to the children. They believed that they were striking at the root of beggary by not allowing it to continue from one generation to another. "Whereas without such regard taken, they may happen to become more poor than their poor parents; and also become evil members, to the great grief of such as daily relieve them in this howse."[92] However, it would also be a mistake to characterize Christ's Hospital as a paradise for needy children. Christ's Hospital was the residence of children who were orphans, foundlings, sick, or disabled, as well as of others who were homeless, destitute, or hungry, regardless of the circumstances of their parents. Christ's Hospital served as a combination of a modern welfare system, foster home, and job retraining camp. The governors of Christ's Hospital created and maintained an institution that is a credit to the compassionate spirit that lives in all of us but fails to find expression often enough. London's children were fortunate that the governors had the courage to act upon that compassion.

Conclusion

As this book has shown, Christ's Hospital was a good place for children—a place where orphans were treated with kindness and compassion. The hospital went beyond merely supplying food, clothing, and shelter; these orphans were given an education and taught a trade. The orphanage was committed to ensuring that their charges would make a successful transition from Christ's to the adult community of London. It was hoped that thus equipped to make a living as adults, those who had been children at Christ's would not continue to be an economic burden on their society but could support themselves and their children.

The orphanage was founded in 1552, along with St. Thomas and Bridewell, to handle the problem of poverty. Their founding was, in some respects, a continuation of the medieval spirit of charity, but it must be kept in mind that sixteenth-century London's response to poverty was fundamentally different from the medieval response. Bridewell, a workhouse, is a good example of the change. Pre-Reformation society basically left charity to the individual's conscience. The poor, or more especially the vagrant, were perceived as embodying the seeds of destruction of a society already vulnerable to breakdown over the great religious issues of the Reformation and the great economic fluctuations of the sixteenth century. Traditionally, people had seen poverty as a benign, pitiable condition that allowed for the exercise of Christian values and a chance to emulate the life of Christ. Medievals could choose to follow a life of poverty: the vow of poverty was one of the oaths sworn by people wanting to assume entry into one of the religious orders. Someone like St. Francis of Assisi, who didn't want the responsibility for the ownership of his own clothes, would have been an enigma to the governing elite of London. If he had wandered into Tudor London, he probably would have wound up in the workhouse of Bridewell. By the sixteenth century in England, religious piety was expressed by contributing money to the poor, not by renouncing material possessions and choosing to live a life of poverty.

As committed as the governors were to running the hospital to the best of their abilities, they were unable to generate enough money to keep Christ's from the threat of bankruptcy. Somehow, the governors managed to keep the hospital in operation. Christ's Hospital, although it has long ceased to be an orphanage, still functions as a school in London today. The legacy of providing an excellent education, started in 1552, still continues today.

Appendix A

A wealth of fiscal information is provided in the two volumes that constitute the Treasurer's Account Books. Only a computerized study can permit analysis of the complicated picture presented by these records of account. All the fiscal analysis contained in chapter 3 on revenues and chapter 4 on expenditures are garnered from computer analysis.

One difficulty in studying the Treasurer's Account Books relates to the problem of converting quantities into meaningful measures; different units were utilized to measure the same commodity. Fish were bought in cades, lasts, hundreds, barrels, and quarters. How many cades or lasts were in a barrel or vice versa is a good question and illustrates the difficulty in reconciling quantities to satify the modern obsession with precision of measurement. Additionally, quantities are difficult to compare because instead of a measurable unit of volume, items were recorded in terms of a unit of time. For example, the sum of money spent for one month on "beef & mutton" in October of 1596 was £12 6s 2d; the actual quantities of either beef or mutton are not recorded.[1]

I have computerized the Treasurer's Account Books, because they contain vital economic information and there is too much contained in the two volumes, totaling over eight hundred pages, to be easily analyzed by hand. My goal in the computerization process was to retain as much information as was revealed in a particular entry. Therefore, very little preselection of data was done. Each line of data generally refers to a single entry in the Treasurer's Account Books. Each entry contains the day, month, year, what the thing was, how much it cost, how much of it there was, what the units were, and whether it was a debit or credit. Although it is a little awkward, I have not altered the spelling of items; this should make it easier to trace specific entries back to the original locale in the Treasurer's Account Books.

However, it is not just their bulk that makes the account books difficult but the manner in which entires were made. The account books give both income and expenditure, but these are not listed in today's bookkeeping style, which makes it possible to tell at a glance the "bottom line." Instead of having debits on one side and credits on the other, the treasurer listed revenues or credits first, usually for a year, and continued until all such items were listed. Then the expenditures were listed, usually for a year, and the list would go on page after page until all entries of expenditure were recorded. Although subtotals are usually entered at the bottom of each page and sometimes certain types of entries were also subtotaled, it is still too cumbersome to tally these numbers in their original format, even accepting that the subtotals are correct. Auditors, who were also governors, were annually appointed to oversee and verify the accuracy of the Treasurer's Account Books.

The third reason that compelled me to use computer analysis is that the numbers are in roman numerals.[2] Adding columns of roman numerals by hand almost guarantees numerous errors, especially as the columns tend to be long. Another factor that complicated the arithmatic is the value of Tudor currency. Twelve pence equals a shilling, twenty shillings equals a pound, and there are also quarter-pence and half-pence, which adds fractions in roman numerals. I have designed, with a consultant, a computer program that allows me to enter figures as roman numerals and the computer then converts them into arabic numerals. The computer converts the pence and shillings into percentages of pounds and then adds them together to get a total for a single entry. For example, twenty shillings would be entered as xxS. and would be recorded as 1.0000 pounds. The reason I decided to enter prices and amounts as roman numerals and have the machine convert them was to avoid the errors that are inherent in conversion on the spot.

Rather than coding the items and entering them in the usual manner historians use, I have a program that allows me to enter items in their original form. Each entry had 9 items: day, month, year, name of the item (itmnam), price, amount of units, units, debit, and credit. For example, the entry "paid the 13th of June 1554 for half a gross of girdles – 16d" would be entered in my program as:

13 06 54 girdle .0300 i halfgross D.[3]

In not having to code all my data, I have saved time and energy by not needing to resort to a codebook to translate variables into names and vice versa.

My program, called "England," issues a prompt at every step before entering data.[4] If I introduce the item name "girdle" for the first time, the program asks me if this is a new entry; if I enter "y" for yes, it adds this to the list in the "itmnam" file. If I enter "n" for no, then the program allows me to reenter or to have the list of itmnam run. The units entry works in the same manner. In this way, "England" protects me from making spelling errors. "England" is the program file and I have three input files: "itmnam," "units," and "alofit." All information in the database is stored in the "alofit" file. The example concerning girdles cited above is the actual entry in "alofit." The "itmnam" file contains all the names of things in each entry. This file contains, for example, milk, cheese, beef, and wool, and holds up to 1,000 names. The "unit" file contains, for example, gallon, yard, year, and month. The "units" file describes units of measurement of either time or quantity. "Alofit" contains 12,184 lines of data and nearly 97,000 variables entered on an IBM mainframe. The chapters on revenues and expenditures are the result of the study of the documents and a statistical study of the database using programs developed specifically for use on this project. The next step was to construct a matrix wherein every item was put into a table by price and year. It proved to be impossible to do the same with the units, because the measurements are imprecise (or in some cases only the name for the measurement is known). This seems to be the nature of the Tudor beast. The Elizabethans had no need for the degree of precision of measurement that has since become standard in the modern world. For example, "a thousand" can mean either a thousand units of something or a simply a large number of something. Billet, which is wood used for fuel, was measured in thousands but this does not mean necessarily that there were a thousand pieces of wood. Moreover, the measurement of a thousand does not make reference to the size of each piece and surely sizes must have varied. Therefore, no two thousands of billet were ever exactly the same. The *Oxford English Dictionary* says "thousand" is "often used vaguely or hyperbolically for a large number. O.E. A thousand of some weight, measure, or quantity."[5]

I took the raw data and aggregated it into 830 groups, which was the same file as the itmnam listing.[6] I then reduced the 830 into the much more manageable number of 28.[7] The last step in analysis of this data was to graph it. All the statistics and the graphs generated from them were produced by the program Lotus 1-2-3.[8]

Appendix B

Governors of the Royal Hospitals

Name	*Guild*	*Hospital*	*Years*	*Sheriff*	*Mayor*
Abraham, William	Vinter	St. Thomas	1576–78		
Ackworth, Thomas	Merchant Tailor	Bridewell	1557–60		
Adams, Richard	Sadler	Christ's	1574–77		
Albany, William	Merchant Tailor	Christ's	1561–63 & 1585–86		
Alden, John	Grocer	St. Bart's	1592–93		
Aldersey, Thomas	Haber- dasher	Christ's Bridewell St. Thomas	1585–96 1574–79 1581–84		
Alderson John	Vintner	St. Thomas	1592–96		
Alison, Robert	Brewer	Christ's	1592–98		
Allen, Thomas	Skinner	Christ's	1566–69 & 1598–99 Bridewell	 1584–85	

Name	*Guild*	*Hospital*	*Years*	*Sheriff*	*Mayor*
Allen, Thomas	Haber-dasher	Bridewell	1580–84		
Allen, Sir Wm.	Skinner	Bridewell St. Thomas	1564–66 1560–63 & 1574–85	1562–53	1571–72
Allen, William	?	Christ's	1592–93		
Allot, Sir John	Fish-monger	Bridewell	1569–79 & 1581–87	1580–81	Part of 1590
Alsoppe, John	Haber-dasher	Bridewell	1577–79 & 1580–82		
Altham, James	Cloth-worker	St. Thomas	1559–60		
Amorie, James	Salter	Christ's	1591–98		
Anderson, Henry	?	St. Bart's	1592–93	1601–2	
Anslowe, William	Skinner	Christ's St. Thomas	1568–75 1559–60 & 1581–87		
Appowell, Robert	Haber-dasher	Christ's	1575–76 & 1580–82		
Archer, John	Fish-monger	St. Thomas	1583–87		
Arnold, Richard	Haber-dasher	Bridewell	1592–93		
Ashby, Richard	Embroiderer	Bridewell	1592–93		
Aske, Robert	Goldsmith	Bridewell	1582–84		
Aske, Robert	Goldsmith	Christ's	1581–82 & 1586–87		

Name	*Guild*	*Hospital*	*Years*	*Sheriff*	*Mayor*
Askewe, John	?	Bridewell	1558–60		
Atkinson, John	Scrivener	Bridewell St. Bart's	1563–64 1557–63		
Atkinson, Thomas	Grocer	Christ's	1566–67		
Atwell, Lawrence	Skinner	St. Bart's	1584–87		
Audley, Thomas	Skinner	Christ's	1570–79 & 1580–87		
Avenon, Sir Alex.	Iron-monger	Christ's Bridewell St. Thomas	1562–68 & 1580–82 1559–61 & 1571–80 1571–73	1561–62	1569–70
Aworthe	?	Bridewell	1558–59		
Aylamer	Cutler	Bridewell	1573–74		
Babham, William	Grocer,	Bridewell	1577–79 & 1580–85		
Backhouse, Nicolas	Grocer	Christ's St. Bart's	1566–71 1574–77		
Bacon, James	Fish-monger	St. Thomas	1559–73	1568–69	
Bacon, Thomas	Salter	Bridewell	1563–64		
Baieworth, Jo	Grocer	Christ's	1596–98		
Baker, John	Mercer	St. Thomas	1561–66		
Baker, Peter	Skinner	St. Thomas	1569–76		

Name	*Guild*	*Hospital*	*Years*	*Sheriff*	*Mayor*
Ballett, John	Goldsmith	Christ's	1593–95		
Band	Haber-dasher	Christ's Bridewell St. Thomas	1576–77 1582–85 1570–71		
Banisted, Roger	Embroiderer	Bridewell	1561–65		
Bankes, Edward	Haber-dasher	Christ's St. Bart's	1556–57 1561–63	1563–64	
Banks, Thomas	Barber-Surgeon	Christ's	1578–98 Interrupt		
Bannester, Thomas	Skinner	St. Bart's Christ's	1564–66 1561–65		
Banning, Paul	Grocer	Christ's	1592–93	1593–94	
Barnes, Bart.	Mercer	Christ's	1592–93 & 1596–97		
Barnes, Sir George	Haber-dasher	St. Bart's St.Thomas Christ's	1567–72 1577–78 & 1580–87 1575–76	1576–77	1586–87
Barnes, John	Leather-seller	Christ's	1578–79 & 1581–85		
Barnes, John	Haber-dasher	St. Thomas	1567–69		
Barnes, Richard	Mercer	St. Bart's	1564–66		
Barnham, Benet	Draper	Christ's	1592–93 & 1595–96	1591–92	
Barnham, Francis	Draper	Bridewell St. Thomas	1559–61 & 1572–74 1562–70 & 1575–76	1570–71	

Name	*Guild*	*Hospital*	*Years*	*Sheriff*	*Mayor*
Barrett, Richard	Mercer	Christ's	1595–99		
Basforde, George	?	Christ's	1560–64		
Bashe, Edward	Cloth-worker	Christ's	1566–68		
Basker-field,	?	St. Thomas	1559–61		
Baskerville, Humfry	Grocer	Christ's Bridewell St. Bart's	1556–57 1559–61 1557–58	1561–62	
Bates, Thomas	Haber-dasher	Christ's St. Thomas	1597–99 1584–85		
Baticks, Thomas	Barber-Surgeon	Christ's	1592–93		
Baudle	Haber-dasher	Christ's	1575–76		
Bawdler, Henry	Draper	Christ's	1586–87		
Bayard, Thomas	Cloth-worker	St. Bart's	1575–78		
Becher, Henry	Haber-dasher	St. Bart's St. Thomas	1567–71 & 1586–87 1580–83	1569–70	
Beckett, Anselm	Haber-dasher	St. Bart's	1576–79 & 1580–81		
Bednam, William	Grocer	Christ's	1594–95		
Benison, Francis	Haber-dasher	St. Thomas	1567–71		
Beswick, William	Draper	St. Bart's	1559–61		

Name	*Guild*	*Hospital*	*Years*	*Sheriff*	*Mayor*
Billingsley, Sir Hugh	Haber- dasher	St.Thomas	1581–87 & 1592–96	1584–85	Part of 1596–97
Bishop, George	Stationer	Christ's	1595–98		
		Bridewell	1592–94		
Bistow, Peter	?	St. Bart's	1560–63		
Blaggs, Michael	Tallow- chandler	St. Thomas	1571–76		
Blanke, Sir Thomas	Haber- dasher?	Bridewell	1581–85	1574–75	1582–83
Blunt, John	Cloth- worker	Christ's	1581–85 & 1592–97		
Blunt, Thomas	Mercer	Bridewell	1573–75		
Blunt, William	Mercer	Christ's	1595–98		
		Bridewell	1572–73		
Boa, Henry	?	St. Bart's	1592–93		
Bodnam, William	Grocer	Christ's	1575–78		
Bond, Anthony	Scrivener	Christ's	1565–66		
Bond, Sir George	Haber- dasher	Bridewell	1581–83 & 1586–92	1578–79	1587–88
		St. Thomas	1570–71		
		Christ's	1575–78		
Bond, Thomas	?	Bridewell	1561–63		
Bonde	?	St. Thomas	1558–59		
Boorne, John	Leather- seller	Christ's	1578–85		

Name	*Guild*	*Hospital*	*Years*	*Sheriff*	*Mayor*
Boreman, Simon	Haber-dasher	Bridewell	1592–93		
Bound, William	Haber-dasher	St. Thomas	1592–93		
Bowes, Sir Mar.	Goldsmith	Bridewell Christ's	1564–66 1559–60	1540–41	1545–46
Box, William	Grocer	Bridewell St. Thomas	1559–63 & 1578–79 1563–64	1570–71	
Boyer, Francis	Grocer	Christ's St. Bart's	1568–72 1578–79 & 1580–81		
Boyer, Redman	?	St. Thomas	1566–67		
Boyer, Reynold	?	Bridewell	1566–67		
Brace, Thomas	Haber-dasher	Bridewell St. Thomas	1572–74 1569–79		
Bradley	?	Bridewell	1557–58		
Bradshaw, Thomas	Mercer	Christ's Bridewell	1562–64 & 1580–81 1566–70 & 1577–79		
Bragg, Edmund	Haber-dasher	Bridewell	1569–57 & 1580–85		
Bramley, Thomas	Haber-dasher	St. Thomas	1581–87		
Branch, John	Draper	Bridewell St. Thomas	1578–79 1557–58 & 1569–70	1571–72	1580–81
Branche	?	Christ's	1558–59		
Brandon, Robert	Goldsmith	Christ's	1581–87		

Name	*Guild*	*Hospital*	*Years*	*Sheriff*	*Mayor*
Braythwate	Draper	St. Thomas	1570–72		
Brecie, Thomas	Haber-dasher	St. Thomas	1569–71 & 1573–74		
Brend	Scrivener	St. Bart's	1570–72		
Brett, Robert	Merchant Tailor	Christ's Bridewell	1582–85 1577–79 & 1580–81		
Bright, Edward	Iron-monger	St. Bart's	1564–73		
Broke, Robert	Grocer	Christ's	1581–87 & 1589–90	1590–91	
Brokebranc William	Grocer	Bridewell	1592–93		
Brokesby, Barchell	Skinner	St. Bart's	1579–75		
Brown	Skinner	Bridewell	1574–76		
Brown, John	Cloth-worker	St. Bart's	1575–77		
Brown, Humphrey	Girdler	St. Thomas	1583–87		
Brown, Thomas	Merchant Tailor	Christ's	1570–76		
Brown, Thomas	Scrivener	Bridewell	1575–76		
Buckland, Richard	?	Christ's Bridewell	1556–58 1562–72		
Buckle, Sir Cut.	Vintner	St. Thomas	1575–78 & 1580–93	1582–83	Part of 1593
Burton, Simon	Wax-chandler	St. Thomas	1573–76		

Name	*Guild*	*Hospital*	*Years*	*Sheriff*	*Mayor*
Bush, Henry	Skinner	Christ's St. Bart's	1556–58 1558–60		
Butler	Haber-dasher	Christ's	1559–61		
Butler, Henry	Draper	Christ's	1559–62		
Cage, Anthony	Salter	Christ's	1573–76 & 1581–82		
Cage, John	Salter	Christ's St. Bart's	1559–64 & 1572–83 1586–87 & 1592–93		
Calthrope, Anthony	Mercer	Christ's	1574–77		
Calthrope, Sir Mar.	Draper	Christ's St. Bart's	1578–79 & 1580–87 1571–75	1579–80	Part of 1588
Cambell, Robert	Iron-monger	St. Thomas	1580–81 & 1592–94		
Cambell, Sir. Thomas	Iron-monger	Christ's	1582–87 & 1592–98	1600–1601	1609–10
Campion, Henry	Mercer	Christ's	1575–78		
Carew, William	Draper	St. Thomas	1583–84		
Carne	Preacher	Bridewell	1580–81		
Cater John	Vintner	St. Thomas	1557–59		
Caverley, Brian	Draper	St. Thomas Bridewell	1583–85 1580–81		
Cennie, Martin	Cloth-worker	Bridewell	1571–73		

Name	*Guild*	*Hospital*	*Years*	*Sheriff*	*Mayor*
Chaire	?	St. Thomas	1560–63		
Chamberlain, Richard	Iron-monger	Christ's St. Bart's	1561–62 1564–66		
Chamberlain, Rol	?	Christ's	1594–98		
Champe	Goldsmith	Christ's	1575–76		
Champion, Sir Ric.	Draper	St. Thomas	1560–65	1558–59	1565–66
Chapman, Edmund	Joiner	St. Thomas	1581–82		
Chapman, John	Tallow-chandler	Christ's	1564–66		
Cheeke, John	Mercer	Bridewell	1580–85		
Chelsam, William	Mercer	Christ's	1566–68		
Chester, Sir W.	Draper	Bridewell St. Thomas	1564–68 1557–63 & 1568–71	1554–55	1560–61
Chevall, William	Draper	Bridewell	1564–65		
Cholsame	Mercer	Christ's	1566–67		
Churchman, John	Merchant Tailor	Bridewell	1582–87		
Clarke, Roger	Salter	Christ's	1586–87 & 1592–93	1599–1600	
Clerk, John	Cloth-worker	Bridewell	1571–79 & 1580–87		
Cluthers, Henry	?	St. Thomas	1592–93		

Name	*Guild*	*Hospital*	*Years*	*Sheriff*	*Mayor*
Cobb, Robert	Grocer?	Bridewell	1592–93		
Cocker, William	Skinner?	Christ's	1573–74		
Cocks, William	?	St. Bart's	1565–66		
Cogan, Robert	Cloth-worker	Christ's St. Bart's	1593–99 1582–87 & 1592–93		
Cokram, Philip	Mercer	Christ's	1584–87		
Coleby, John	Cloth-worker?	Christ's	1598–99		
Colecloth, Mathew	Draper	Bridewell St. Thomas	1570–74 1574–78		
Coles, William	Grocer	St. Bart's	1580–85		
Colethurst, H.	Grocer	St. Bart's	1592–94		
Colett, Richard	?	St. Bart's	1584–85		
Colmer, Richard	Grocer	Christ's	1577–79		
Colmere, John	Grocer	Bridewell	1580–81		
Colson, Gabriel	Grocer	Bridewell St. Bart's	1577–79 1581–84		
Colston	?	St. Thomas	1561–62		
Colverwell, Ric	Mercer	St. Bart's	1583–86		
Cooper	Grocer	Christ's St. Thomas	1568–69 1570–71		

Name	*Guild*	*Hospital*	*Years*	*Sheriff*	*Mayor*
Cooper, Richard	Dyer	Christ's St. Thomas	1589–94 1573–75		
Cordall, Thomas	Mercer	Christ's	1592–93		
Cornhill, Thomas	Fish-monger	St. Thomas	1564–65		
Cotts	?	St. Thomas	1562–63		
Couche	Innholder	Bridewell	1581–83		
Coxe, William	Haber-dasher	St. Bart's	1564–66		
Coxe, William	Grocer	St. Thomas	1565–75		
Cranefeld, Thomas	Mercer	Christ's	1573–76		
Craven, Sir William	Merchant Tailor	Christ's	1594–97	1600–1601	1610–11
Crender	Vintner	Christ's Bridewell	1581–82 1575–78		
Crouch, Richard	Sadler	Bridewell	1592–94		
Crowther, George	Vintner	Bridewell	1577–78 & 1580–82		
Cupper	?	Christ's	1595–97		
Cure, Thomas	Sadler	Bridewell	1580–85		
Dabb, Henry	Haber-dasher	St. Bart's	1578–79		
Dale, Henry	Haber-dasher	Bridewell St. Bart's	1580–87 1577–78		
Dane, William	Iron-monger	Christ's St. Bart's	1556–58 1558–60	1569–70	

Name	*Guild*	*Hospital*	*Years*	*Sheriff*	*Mayor*
Danster Thomas	Girdler	St. Bart's	1580–85		
Dawbrey, Arthur	Merchant Tailor	Bridewell St. Bart's	1575–79 1557–58		
Denham, William	Goldsmith	Christ's Bridewell St. Thomas	1576–79 1571–73 1595–96		
Dent, John	?	Christ's	1587–88		
Derham, Baldwin	Mercer	Christ's	1583–86 & 1589–96		
Deuckes	Grocer	Christ's	1570–71		
Dichefeld, Thomas	Salter	St. Thomas	1557–60		
Dickenson, Robert	Draper	Bridewell	1572–74 & 1580–83		
Dixie, Sir Wolstane	Skinner	Christ's Bridewell	1573–75 & 1580–93 1570–71 & 1576–77	1575–76	1585–86
Dixson	Goldsmith	Bridewell	1573–74		
Dixson, Thomas	Cloth-worker	Christ's	1573–74		
Dixson, Thomas	Skinner	Christ's	1572–74		
Dobbs, John	Skinner	Bridewell	1573–75		
Dodd, Francis	Haber-dasher	Bridewell	1576–79		
Dodd, George	Vintner	Bridewell	1583–85		

Name	*Guild*	*Hospital*	*Years*	*Sheriff*	*Mayor*
Dodworth. William	Merchant Tailor	St. Bart's	1580–87 & 1592–93		
Dormar, William	?	Bridewell	1592–93		
Dorrel	Merchant Tailor	St. Bart's	1580–81		
Douckens	Merchant Tailor	Christ's	1570–71		
Dove, Edward	?	Bridewell	1561–63		
Draper, Sir Charles	Iron-monger	St. Thomas	1557–66 & 1573–79	1560–61	1566–67
Drew	Recorder	Bridewell	1592–93		
Ducket, Sir Lionel	Mercer	Christ's Bridewell St. Thomas	1556–60 1566–85 1573–74	1564–65	1572–73
Dykers	?	St. Bart's	1559–60		
Edmonds, John	Fish-monger	Bridewell St. Thomas	1592–93 1577–78		
Edwards, Christopher	Haber-dasher	Christ's	1564–71		
Edwards, John	Vintner	St. Thomas	1592–93		
Egerton, Thomas	Mercer	Christ's	1582–89		
Elkin, William	Mercer	Christ's	1578–93	1586–87	
Elmer, Edward	Grocer	Christ's	1573–76		
Eorste, Robert	Iron-monger	Christ's	1580–81		

Name	*Guild*	*Hospital*	*Years*	*Sheriff*	*Mayor*
Esling, Henry	Baker	St. Bart's	1566–73		
Eyland, Mathew	Cutler	Bridewell	1565–74		
Fairfax, Humphrey	Grocer	Bridewell	1577–78		
Falkenstein, Richard	Skinner	St. Thomas	1573–74		
Farrington, Richard	Cloth-worker	Christ's	1596–99		
Fawks, Henry	Grocer	Bridewell	1582–87		
Fetiplace, Theodore	Iron-monger	Bridewell	1590–93		
Fiche, Randolph	Vintner	Christ's	1592–93		
Field, Mathew	Mercer	Christ's	1570–73		
Fish, Cornelius	Skinner	St. Bart's	1595–96		
Fish, Walter	Merchant Tailor	Christ's Bridewell	1577–78 & 1581–82 1580–81		
Fisher, Thomas	Skinner	Christ's	1596–99		
Flecton, Robert	Grocer	Christ's	1556–58		
Fleetwood, William	Recorder	Bridewell	1580–87		
Fletcher, William	Skinner	Christ's St. Bart's	1556–58 1558–59		

Name	*Guild*	*Hospital*	*Years*	*Sheriff*	*Mayor*
Forman, George	Skinner	Christ's	1575–76		
Fowler, Edward	Grocer	St. Bart's	1559–61		
Fowlkes, Richard	Cloth-worker	Christ's	1575–71		
Fox	Goldsmith	Bridewell	1580–81		
France, Henry	Grocer	Bridewell	1581–82		
Fulkheath	Skinner	Bridewell	1583–84		
Gamage, Anthony	Iron-monger	Christ's	1562–64 & 1573–79	1574–75	
		Bridewell	1568–73		
Gannell, James	Stationer	St. Bart's	1586–87		
Gardener, Thomas	Goldsmith	Christ's	1561–65		
		Bridewell	1565–69 & 1573–76		
Gardiner, John	Mercer	Christ's	1596–99		
Garrard, Anthony	Mercer	Christ's	1576–79		
		St. Bart's	1585–87		
		St. Thomas	1595–96		
Garrard, Sir William	Haber-dasher	St. Bart's	1559–72 & 1595–96	1552–53	1555–56
		Bridewell	1557–59		
Garrett, Sir John	Haber-dasher	St. Thomas	1582–84 & 1586–87	1592–93	1601–2
Garten, Giles	Iron-monger	St. Thomas	1580–85		
		Christ's	1587–88		

Name	*Guild*	*Hospital*	*Years*	*Sheriff*	*Mayor*
Gibbons, William	Salter	Bridewell	1561–64 & 1577–78		
		St. Bart's	1568–75		
		Christ's	1580–81		
Gilbert	?	Bridewell	1561–63		
Gilbert, Henry	Goldsmith	St. Bart's	1557–58		
Gilborne	Cloth-worker	St. Thomas	1580–81		
Glover, Sir William	Dyer	Christ's	1595–99		
		Bridewell	1592–93		
Goldbee	?	Christ's	1598–99		
Golstone, Gabriel	Grocer	Bridewell	1577–78		
		St. Bart's	1580–81		
Golstone, Richard	Salter	St. Thomas	1561–65		
Gore, Thomas	Grocer	St. Bart's	1564–67		
Grafton, Richard	Grocer	Christ's	1552–63		
		Bridewell	1557–61		
Green	Girdler	St. Thomas	1572–73		
Green, Lawrence	Cutler	Bridewell	1567–68		
		St. Thomas	1573–81		
Greenway, Ralph	Grocer	St. Thomas	1557–58		
Gresham, Sir John	Mercer	Christ's	1567–70	1537–38	1547–48
Gunter, Philip	Skinner	St. Thomas	1575–78 & 1580–81		
Gurney, Richard	Haber-dasher	Christ's	1586–87 & 1592–96		

Name	*Guild*	*Hospital*	*Years*	*Sheriff*	*Mayor*
Hager, William	Salter	Bridewell	1565–71		
Haidnye	Cloth-worker	St. Bart's	1581–82		
Hale, Richard	Grocer	St. Bart's	1581–87 & 1592–93		
Hall	Draper	Bridewell	1580–81		
Hall, Edward	Haber-dasher	St. Thomas	1564–66 & 1573–75		
Hall, Edward	Wood-monger	Bridewell	1586–87		
Hall, Richard	Merchant Tailor	Christ's	1574–77		
Hall, Thomas	Salter	Christ's St. Bart's	1574–82 1566–74		
Hampson, Sir Robert	Merchant Tailor	St. Bart's	1592–93 & 1595–96	1598–99	
Handberie, William	Baker	St. Thomas	1592–93		
Harding, John	Salter	St. Bart's St. Thomas	1564–70 1573–77		
Harding, Robert	Salter	Christ's Bridewell St. Thomas	1558–62 & 1570–71 1560–68 1557–58		
Harding, William	Cloth-worker	Christ's St. Bart's	1569–70 1581–82		
Hare, William	Leather-seller	Bridewell St. Bart's	1567–69 1557–58		
Harper, Sir William	Merchant Tailor	Christ's St. Bart's	1559–60 1552–53	1556–57	1561–62
Harris, Sir James	?	Bridewell	1577–78		

Name	*Guild*	*Hospital*	*Years*	*Sheriff*	*Mayor*
Harris, Robert	?	Bridewell	1559–65		
Harrison, James	Goldsmith	Bridewell	1563–64 & 1569–70		
Harrison, John	Goldsmith	Christ's	1556–58 & 1580–81		
Hart, Sir John	Grocer	St. Bart's Bridewell	1570–79 & 1584–93	1579–80	1589–90
Harvey	?	Christ's	1560–61		
Harvey, James	Iron-monger	St. Thomas	1570–73	1573–74	1581–82
Harvey, John	Skinner	St. Bart's St. Thomas Bridewell	1584–87 1593–94 1580–81		
Hastewe, John	?	Bridewell	1557–59		
Haulse	?	St. Bart's	1557–58		
Hawes, Sir James	Cloth-worker	Christ's Bridewell St. Bart's	1562–63 & 1566–75 1576–81 1563–64	1565–66	1574–75
Hawes, Robert	Merchant Tailor	Christ's	1583–99		
Hawkins, Paul	Vintner	Christ's	1597–99		
Hayden, John	Mercer	Christ's	1577–82	1582–83	
Hayley, Richard	Grocer	St. Bart's	1582–86		
Hayward, John	Draper	Bridewell St. Thomas	1557–62 1558–60		

Name	*Guild*	*Hospital*	*Years*	*Sheriff*	*Mayor*
Hayward, Sir Row.	Cloth-worker	Bridewell St. Bart's Christ's	1562–66 1572–93 1561–93 Interrupt	1563–64	1570–71 1590
Hearson, Thomas	Draper	St. Thomas	1577–78		
Heath, Stephen	Cooper	St. Thomas	1557–70		
Heaton, Francis	Goldsmith	Christ's	1577–79		
Heaton, Thomas	Mercer	Christ's	1559–61 & 1568–70		
Henley, Hugh	Merchant Tailor	Bridewell	1583–87		
Hewes, James	Grocer	Christ's Bridewell	1582–86 1577–79		
Hewet, Henry	Cloth-worker	St. Thomas	1580–83		
Hewet, Sir Thomas	Cloth-worker	St. Thomas	1561–63		
Hewet, Sir William	Cloth-worker	St. Bart's St. Thomas	1575–81 1561–67	1553–54	1559–60
Hewson, Richard	Skinner	St. Thomas	1586–87		
Higgens, Anthony	Skinner	Bridewell	1573–74		
Highlord, John	Skinner	Christ's	1586–99		
Hill, Sir Rowland	Mercer	Bridewell	1557–62	1541–42	1549–50
Hilliard, John	Goldsmith	Christ's	1580–82		

Name	*Guild*	*Hospital*	*Years*	*Sheriff*	*Mayor*
Hills, John	Skinner	St. Bart's	1584–87		
Hills, Richard	Merchant Tailor	Christ's	1570–76		
Hilson, Robert	Mercer	Christ's Bridewell St. Bart's	1576–84 1557–61 1561–64		
Hobson, William	Haber-dasher	Christ's Bridewell	1576–79 1567–68		
Hogeson, William	Merchant Tailor	Christ's	1573–75		
Hoggs, Thomas	Haber-dasher	St. Thomas	1573–74		
Hole	Fishmonger	Christ's	1582–87		
Holiday, Sir Leo	Merchant Tailor	Bridewell	1592–93	1595–96	1605–6
Holmeden, Edward	Grocer	Christ's	1592–93		
Horne, William	Grocer	Bridewell	1584–87		
Horsepoole, Simon	Clothier	Christ's	1593–94 & 1596–97		
Hoskins, Charles	Merchant Tailor	Christ's	1578–82		
House, Robert	Cloth-worker	St. Bart's	1573–79	1586–87	
Howland	?	St. Bart's Christ's	1563–64		
Hughes, James	Grocer	Bridewell	1577–78		
Hunt	Leather-seller	Bridewell	1568–69		

Name	*Guild*	*Hospital*	*Years*	*Sheriff*	*Mayor*
Hunt, Thomas	Fish-monger	Bridewell	1592–93		
Huntley, Humfrey	Iron-monger	Christ's	1586–97		
Huntocke, Henry	Merchant Tailor	St. Bart's	1586–87		
Ireland, John	Salter	Bridewell	1592–93		
Isboard, Godfrey	Haber-dasher	Bridewell	1580–95		
Isham, Henry	Mercer	Christ's	1580–95		
Jackman, Edward	Grocer	Bridewell St. Bart's St. Thomas	1557–59 1562–64 1566–68	1564–65	
Jackman, John	Grocer	St. Bart's	1585–87		
Jackson, John	?	Christ's	1561–74		
Janyners	Draper	St. Thomas	1565–66		
Jeff	?	Bridewell	1570–71		
Jennyns, Thomas	Leather-seller	Christ's Bridewell	1557–65 1565–67		
Johnson, Thomas	Skinner	Christ's	1561–63		
Jones, Roger	Dyer	St. Bart's	1592–93 & 1595–96		
Judde, Sir Andrew	Goldsmith	Christ's	1556–58	1544–45	1550–51
Katcher, John	Pewterer	Bridewell	1593–94	1587–88	

Name	*Guild*	*Hospital*	*Years*	*Sheriff*	*Mayor*
Keale, Hugh	Goldsmith	Christ's St. Bart's	1561–64 1592–93 & 1595–96		
Kelk, Clement	Haber-dasher	Bridewell	1573–79 & 1581–84		
Kempton, Edward	Merchant Tailor	Christ's Bridewell	1592–93 1569–76		
Kempton, William	Merchant Tailor	Christ's	1594–96	1576–77	
Key	?	Christ's	1594–96		
King, John	Tallow-chandler	Christ's	1559–73		
King, Warner	Fish-monger	Bridewell	1592–93		
King, William	Grocer	Christ's	1560–64 & 1571–72		
Kirby, John	Grocer	Christ's	1574–78		
Kythley, Thomas	Leather-seller	Bridewell	1561–66		
Lacy, John	Cloth-worker	Bridewell St. Bart's	1562–68 1580–86		
Lambe, William	Cloth-worker	Christ's	1571–79		
Lambert, Richard	Grocer	Christ's St. Bart's	1564–66 1559–61	1566–67	
Langley, Sir John	Goldsmith	Christ's	1556–57	1566–67	1576–77
Langley, William	Grocer	Bridewell	1568–73		
Laurence, Thomas	Goldsmith	Christ's	1585–93 Interrupt		

Name	*Guild*	*Hospital*	*Years*	*Sheriff*	*Mayor*
Lawes, Robert	Merchant Tailor	Christ's	1592–93		
Lee, Henry	?	Bridewell St. Bart's	1559–61 1562–63		
Leigh, Sir Thomas	Mercer	Bridewell St. Bart's Christ's	1557–60 1561–64 1557–58 & 1562–63	1555–56	
Leners	?	St. Bart's	1557–58		
Leonard, John	Mercer	Christ's	1564–65		
Leonard, William	Mercer	Christ's	1565–69 & 1573–74		
Lethar, William	Cleric	Bridewell	1592–93		
Leveson, William	Mercer	St. Thomas	1592–93		
Lewsam	?	Christ's	1597–98		
Lodge, Sir Thomas	Grocer	St. Thomas	1560–61	1559–60	1562–63
Longe, Morris	Cloth-worker	Christ's	1564–66		
Lorimer, William	Innholder	St. Thomas	1561–64		
Lowe, Nicholas	Merchant Tailor	St. Thomas	1563–68		
Lowe, Thomas	Vintner	St. Bart's	1561–64		
Lowe, Sir Thomas	Haber-dasher	Christ's	1594–95	1595–96	1604–5

Name	*Guild*	*Hospital*	*Years*	*Sheriff*	*Mayor*
Lucas, John	Skinner	Bridewell	1582–87		
Luddington, Nicolas	Grocer	Bridewell St. Bart's	1580–87 1567–68		
Lute, John	Cloth-worker	St. Bart's	1561–64		
Luyer, Francis	Grocer	Christ's	1569–70		
Lynford, William	Merchant Tailor	Bridewell	1592–93		
Lyon, Sir John	Grocer	St. Bart's	1557–58	1550–51	1554–55
Lyslie, Richard	Cloth-worker	Christ's	1567–68		
Lyvers	?	Christ's	1558–59		
Mabbe, John	Goldsmith	Christ's Bridewell	1560–62 1570–78		
Machil, John	Cloth-worker	Christ's	1556–58	1555–56	
Maghow, Richard	Skinner	Christ's	1570–71		
Malory, Sir Richard	Merchant Tailor	Bridewell St. Bart's	1566–67 1558–61	1557–58	1564–65
Manning, Randall	Skinner	Christ's	1591–99		
Marbye, Arthur	Fish-monger	St. Thomas	1575–78		
Marler, Christian	Merchant Tailor	St. Bart's	1566–69 & 1593–94		
Marsh, John	Mercer	Bridewell	1557–60		

Name	*Guild*	*Hospital*	*Years*	*Sheriff*	*Mayor*
Marsh, Robert	Grocer	Christ's	1593–95		
Marston, James	Vintner	Christ's Bridewell	1561–65 1565–68		
Martin, Mathew	Brewer	St. Bart's	1592–93		
Martin, Richard	?	Christ's	1584–87		
Martin, Sir Richard	Goldsmith	Christ's St. Bart's	1560–65 1565–67	1581–82	1588–89 1593–94
Martin, Sir Roger	Mercer	Bridewell	1557–59		
Martin, Roland	?	Christ's	1595–96		
Masham, William	Grocer	St. Bart's	1578–79 & 1580–93	1583–84	
Maston	?	Christ's	1561–62		
Maughan	Skinner	Christ's	1571–72		
Maye, Richard	Merchant Tailor	St. Bart's	1578–79 & 1580–83		
Medcalf, Thomas	Goldsmith	St. Thomas	1559–61		
Meggs, William	Draper	St. Thomas	1576–87 & 1592–93		
Mills, Henry	Grocer	Bridewell	1564–65		
Mills, Leonard	Haber-dasher	Bridewell	1592–94		
More, John	Skinner	Bridewell	1592–94	1597–98	

Name	*Guild*	*Hospital*	*Years*	*Sheriff*	*Mayor*
Morgan, Hugh	Grocer	Christ's	1572–97		
Morris, Richard	?	St. Thomas	1561–66		
Morris, Richard	Iron-monger	Christ's St. Thomas	1580–82 1561–70		
Mosley, Sir Nicolas	Cloth-worker	St. Bart's	1586–87 & 1592–96	1590–91	1599–1600
Muchampe	Goldsmith	Christ's	1576–77		
Mynoures, Richard	Draper	St. Thomas	1560–67		
Newman, Gabriel	Joiner	Bridewell	1586–87 & 1592–94		
Newman, John	Grocer	St. Bart's	1582–87 & 1592–96		
Nicholas, Sir Amb.	Salter	St. Bart's	1558–78	1566–67	1575–76
Norton, William	Stationer	Christ's	1580–94		
Nylby, William	Dyer	St. Thomas	1567–68		
Nylson	Dyer	St. Thomas	1566–67		
Offley, Hugh	Leather-seller	St. Thomas	1575–85 & 1592–93	1588–89	
Offley, Robert	Haber-dasher	Christ's St. Thomas	1558–64 1566–78 & 1580–87		
Offley, Sir Thomas	Merchant Tailor	Christ's	1559–82	1553–54	1556–57
Offley, Thomas	?	Bridewell	1558–59 & 1564–70		

Name	*Guild*	*Hospital*	*Years*	*Sheriff*	*Mayor*
Oldham, John	Cloth-worker	Bridewell	1586–87		
Oleffe, John	Merchant Tailor	St. Thomas	1558–61 & 1566–67	1568–69	
Olive, John	Merchant Tailor	St. Thomas	1563–67 &	1576–77	
Olsinge	Baker	St. Bart's	1566–67		
Onslowe, William	Scrivener	St. Thomas	1558–59 & 1581–82		
Orenshawe, William	Vintner or Grocer	Bridewell	1575–76		
Osborne	Goldsmith	Christ's	1565–66		
Osborne, Sir Edward	Cloth-worker	St. Thomas	1571–75 & 1581–87	1575–76	
Ounstone, William	Skinner	St. Thomas	1576–81 & 1592–93		
Owards	Haberdasher	Bridewell	1569–70		
Owfield	Fishmonger	Christ's	1597–99		
Oxmashouse, W.	Grocer	Bridewell	1576–79		
Paine, Robert	Grocer	Christ's	1592–93		
Palmer, Andrew	Goldsmith	Christ's	1574–96 Interrupt		
Parr, John	Embroiderer	Bridewell	1592–93		
Parson	?	Christ's	1564–65		
Partridge	Goldsmith	Christ's	1574–76		
Peacock, Richard	Leather-seller	Bridewell	1568–71		

Name	*Guild*	*Hospital*	*Years*	*Sheriff*	*Mayor*
Pearson, Thomas	Scrivener	St. Thomas	1557–69		
Pearson, William	Scrivener	Christ's	1557–67		
Peirson, Nicholas	Skinner	St. Bart's	1592–94		
Pelsannt, John	Grocer	Bridewell	1580–85		
Pemberton, Sir James	Goldsmith	Christ's	1594–99	1602–3	1611–12
Pers	?	St. Thomas	1561–62		
Pierce, John	Fish-monger	Bridewell	1560–64		
Pigott, Edmond	Grocer	St. Bart's	1592–93		
Pipe	Leatherseller	Christ's	1568–70		
Pipe, Sir Richard	Draper	Christ's Bridewell	1569–70 1562–63 & 1573–81	1572–73	1578–79
Plasden, William	Iron-monger	St. Thomas	1580–83		
Platt, Richard	Brewer	St. Bart's	1580–87 & 1592–96		
Plummer, Walter?	Merchant Tailor?	Christ's	1598–99		
Pope, Thomas	Merchant Tailor	St. Bart's	1582–87		
Porter, John?	Fish-monger?	Christ's	1595–99 Interrupt		
Powell, Robert	Haber-dasher	Christ's	1575–79 & 1595–97		

Name	*Guild*	*Hospital*	*Years*	*Sheriff*	*Mayor*
Pranell, Henry	Vintner	Christ's	1578–79 & 1580–87	1585–86	
Pratt, Charles	?	St. Thomas	1568–71		
Proctor, Richard	Merchant Tailor	Christ's	1589–99		
Pryor, Anthony	Draper	Christ's	1576–77		
Puell	?	Christ's	1581–82		
Pullison, Sir Thomas	Draper	Christ's	1570–79 & 1580–86	1573–74	1584–85
		Bridewell	1586–88		
Punte	Merchant Tailor	Bridewell	1580–81		
Pygott, John	Grocer	Bridewell	1559–61		
Pynson, Nicholas	Cloth-worker	Bridewell	1578–79		
Quarles, John	Draper	Christ's	1569–70		
Quarles, William	Mercer	Christ's	1557–60 & 1570–75		
		St. Bart's	1592–93		
Queenie, Bartholomew	Cloth-worker	Bridewell	1592–93		
Radcliff, Anthony	Merchant Tailor	Christ's	1576–79 & 1586–87	1585–86	
		Bridewell	1580–81 & 1591–94		
Ramsey, Sir Thomas	Grocer	Christ's	1582–87	1567–68	1577–78
Randall, Vincent	Mercer	Christ's	1561–63		

Name	*Guild*	*Hospital*	*Years*	*Sheriff*	*Mayor*
Redman	Brewer?	St. Thomas	1566–67		
Reynolds	?	Bridewell	1565–67		
Reynolds, Richard	Draper	St. Thomas	1567–74		
Rich, John	Grocer	Bridewell	1578–79		
Ridley	?	Christ's	1596–97		
Riggs, Thomas	Haber-dasher	St. Thomas	1570–78 & 1580–87		
Rivers, Sir John	Grocer	Christ's St. Thomas	1571–73 1576–78 & 1582–84	1565–66	1573–74
Robinson, Francis	Grocer	Christ's	1567–69		
Robinson, William	Barber-Surgeon	Bridewell	1592–93		
Rogers, John	Grocer	St. Thomas	1586–87		
Rogers, Robert	Leather-seller	Christ's	1595–99		
Rose, Robert	Merchant Tailor	Bridewell	1564–69		
Rowe, Henry	Mercer?	St. Bart's	1585–87 & 1592–96	1597–98	1607–8
Rowe, Oliver	Merchant Tailor	Christ's	1582–87		
Rowe, Sir Thomas	Merchant Tailor	St. Thomas	1566–68	1560–61	1568–69
Rowe, Sir William	Iron-monger	Bridewell	1575–76 & 1583–94	1582–83	1592–93

Name	*Guild*	*Hospital*	*Years*	*Sheriff*	*Mayor*
Roxe	?	St. Thomas	1562–63		
Royse, John	Mercer	Christ's	1556–57		
Russell	Haberdasher	Christ's	1559–60		
Russell, Thomas	Draper	St. Thomas	1583–87		
Ryder, Sir William	Haber-dasher	Bridewell	1592–94	1591–92	1600–1601
Ryvell, Nicholas	Grocer	St. Thomas	1569–71		
Saltenstall, Sir Richard	Skinner	Christ's St. Thomas	1583–94 1571–78	1588–89	1597–98
Sanders, Blaise	Grocer	Christ's St. Bart's	1574–76 1577–78		
Sares, Thomas	Haber-dasher	St. Thomas Bridewell	1570–73 1580–81		
Saule, Robert	Salter	Christ's	1577–78		
Sawell, Thomas	Salter	Bridewell	1592–93		
Sawle	?	St. Bart's	1563–64		
Sawyer	?	St. Thomas	1557–63		
Saxson	?	Bridewell	1593–94		
Scoreie	?	Christ's	1593–94		
Scott, John	Salter	St. Bart's	1560–64 & 1572–79		
Sherrington, William	Haber-dasher	Bridewell St. Bart's	1580–87 1569–79		
Sheteham, Thomas	Merchant Tailor	St. Thomas	1567–69		

Name	*Guild*	*Hospital*	*Years*	*Sheriff*	*Mayor*
Shreve, Lawrence	Grocer	Christ's	1565–67		
Silver, Anthony	Leather-seller	Bridewell	1558–61		
Skales, Richard	Salter	Bridewell	1592–93		
Skinner, Oliver	Salter	Bridewell	1592–93		
Skinner, Thomas	Cloth-worker	Christ's	1593–96	1587–88	Part of 1596
Skydmore Steven	Vintner	Christ's Bridewell	1582–85 1575–76		
Slany, Sir Stephen	Skinner	Christ's Bridewell St. Bart's	1582–99 1574–75 & 1580–81 1573–74	1584–85	1595–96
Sleiford, Richard	Cloth-worker	Christ's	1590–93		
Smith, Ambrose	Mercer	Christ's Bridewell	1574–75 1578–79		
Smith, David	Embroiderer	Bridewell	1583–87		
Smith, Gregory	Merchant Tailor	Christ's	1591–94		
Smith, John	Mercer	Christ's	1592–95		
Smith Richard	Mercer	Bridewell	1575–76		
Smith, Sir Thomas	Haber-dasher	St. Bart's	1596–97	1600–1601	
Smythe, Richard	Fish-monger	Bridewell	1575–76		

Name	*Guild*	*Hospital*	*Years*	*Sheriff*	*Mayor*
Sole, Robert	Salter	Christ's St. Bart's	1578–85 1561–62		
Some, Sir Stephen	Grocer	Christ's	1592–93	1589–90	1598–99
Sonne, William	?	Christ's St. Bart's	1556–57 1557–58		
Sotherton, George	Merchant Tailor	Christ's Bridewell St. Bart's	1591–95 1580–85 1585–86		
Sotherton, Now.	Merchant Tailor	St. Bart's	1592–94		
South	Innholder	Bridewell	1580–81		
Southall, John	Cloth-worker	Christ's	1574–87		
Sparke, John	Merchant Tailor	Christ's	1564–69		
Spencer, Sir John	Cloth-worker	St. Bart's St. Thomas	1592–93 1576–78 & 1592–93	1583–84	1594–95
Springham, Richard	Mercer	St. Thomas	1559–63		
Springton	Haberdasher	St. Bart's	1571–72		
Standlake, Anthony	Mercer?	Christ's	1597–99		
Staper, Richard	Cloth-worker	St. Thomas	1592–93		
Starkie, Thomas	Skinner	Bridewell	1568–78 & 1580–87	1578–79	
Stockmeade, George	Grocer	Christ's	1576–79		
Stone, John	Haber-dasher	Christ's Bridewell	1581–82 1592–93		

Name	*Guild*	*Hospital*	*Years*	*Sheriff*	*Mayor*
Stone, William	Haber-dasher	Christ's	1580–82		
Stoorer, John	Baker	Christ's	1585–99		
Store	?	Christ's	1584–85		
Style, Edmund	Grocer	Christ's St. Bart's	1556–57 1557–58		
Sutton, Henry	Goldsmith	Christ's Bridewell	1564–66 1570–71		
Swaldell, Christopher	Barber-Surgeon	Bridewell	1592–97		
Swingfield, Stephen	Fish-monger	Bridewell	1592–93		
Tatt, John	Draper	St. Thomas Christ's	1576–77 & 1581–83		
Taylor, Henry	Cloth-worker	Bridewell	1580–87		
Taylor John	Haber-dasher	Christ's	1592–96		
Taylor, Richard	Grocer?	Bridewell	1561–63		
Taylor Robert	Haber-dasher	St. Thomas	1586–87 & 1592–93	1592–93	
Taylor, Thomas	Goldsmith	Bridewell	1580–87		
Thornhill, Richard	Grocer	Bridewell	1566–70		
Thowgood	Draper	Christ's	1576–79		
Thwaites, William	Fish-monger	Christ's	1592–98		

Name	*Guild*	*Hospital*	*Years*	*Sheriff*	*Mayor*
Tomlinson, Thomas	Skinner	Christ's	1589–99		
Towerson, William	Skinner	Christ's	1578–79 & 1580–82		
Traves, John	Merchant Tailor	Bridewell	1569–70		
Trotte, John	Draper	Christ's	1580–82		
Tues, William	Skinner	Bridewell	1576–77		
Turnebull, Thomas	Haber-dasher	St. Thomas	1564–65		
Velste	Skinner	Bridewell	1570–71		
Venables, Richard	Merchant Tailor	St. Bart's	1592–96		
Vikers	?	St. Bart's	1558–61		
Violet, Richard	Fish-monger	St. Thomas	1561–64		
Vnlok	Draper	St. Thomas	1575–76		
Vydwell, William	Merchant Tailor	Bridewell	1577–78 & 1586–87		
Wade, Thomas	Iron-monger	Christ's Bridewell	1591–99 1580–83		
Wade, Thomas	Pewterer	St. Thomas	1586–87		
Wager	Preacher	Bridewell	1580–87		
Walkeden, Geoffrey	Skinner	Bridewell	1570–72 & 1577–79		
Walker, John	?	Christ's	1593–94		

Name	*Guild*	*Hospital*	*Years*	*Sheriff*	*Mayor*
Walker, Thomas	Vintner	Christ's	1592–93		
Wallis	?	St. Bart's	1558–59		
Walter, Richard	Girdler?	St. Thomas	1586–87		
Ward, John	Leather-seller	Bridewell	1592–93		
Ware, Thomas	Fish-monger	Christ's St. Thomas	1584–87 & 1592–93 1568–73 & 1577–78		
Warfield, Roger	Grocer	Bridewell	1577–79 & 1580–92		
Warner, Nicholas	Skinner	Bridewell	1592–93		
Warthall, Anthony	Mercer	Bridewell Christ's	1592–93 1580–81	1606–7	
Waste, Christopher	Goldsmith	St. Bart's	1592–96		
Wattes, Sir Joseph	Cloth-worker	Christ's	1594–95	1596–97	1606–7
Wayde	?	Bridewell	1593–94		
Waye, Thomas	Vintner	St. Thomas	1580–87		
Weaver, John	Mercer	Bridewell	1592–93		
Webb, Thomas	Haber-dasher	St. Bart's	1595–96		
Webbe, Henry	Merchant Tailor	Bridewell	1586–87		

Name	*Guild*	*Hospital*	*Years*	*Sheriff*	*Mayor*
Webbe, Sir William	Salter	St. Bart's Bridewell	1574–87 & 1592–93 1594–98	1581–82	1591–92
Weld, Nicholas	Draper	St. Thomas	1574–75		
Welke, William	?	St. Bart's	1583–84		
Wells	Scrivener	St. Thomas	1563–64		
Wethens, Lawrence	Salter	Christ's St. Bart's St. Thomas	1560–73 1557–58 1558–60	1553–54	1559–60
Wheeler, Nicholas	Draper	Bridewell St. Thomas	1561–64 1573–74		
White	Preacher	Bridewell	1580–82		
White, John	Haber-dasher	Christ's	1581–84		
White, Sir John	Grocer	Bridewell St. Bart's	1568–72 1557–61 & 1570–71	1556–57	1563–64
White, Ralph	?	St. Thomas	1557–58		
White, Sir Thomas	Merchant Tailor	Christ's	1556–67	1547–48	1553–54
Whitehorn, Joseph	Cloth-worker	Christ's	1560–63		
Whithernes	?	Christ's	1561–62		
Whitmore, William	Haber-dasher	Christ's	1581–85 & 1592–93		
Whitt, Dr.	Cleric	Bridewell	1592–93		
Wiggs, Robert	Goldsmith	Christ's	1562–64		

Name	*Guild*	*Hospital*	*Years*	*Sheriff*	*Mayor*
Wight, John	Draper	Christ's	1582–85		
Wild	?	Christ's	1598–99		
Wilford, Thomas	Merchant Tailor	Christ's Bridewell	1594–95 1589–90		
Wilson	Dyer	St. Thomas	1566–67		
Winche, Robert	Haber-dasher	Bridewell	1574–82		
Wistman, Richard	Goldsmith	Christ's	1594–97		
Withens, Robert	Vintner	St. Thomas	1580–87 & 1592–93		
Witton, Thomas	Scrivener	St. Bart's	1562–70		
Woer, Richard	Dyer	St. Bart's	1592–93		
Woodcock, Hugh	Salter	Bridewell	1592–93		
Woodcock, Ralph	Grocer	Christ's St. Thomas	1572–76 & 1581–86 1577–78		
Woodroffe, Sir Nicholas	Haber-dasher	Bridewell St. Thomas	1578–79 & 1581–83 1567–77 & 1580–85	1572–73	1579–80
Wright, Richard	Iron-monger	Christ's Bridewell	1581–83 & 1595–96 1592–93		
Wyate	Wood-monger?	St. Bart's	1557–58		
Wygnell, Wiliam	Merchant Tailor	Bridewell	1576–77		

Name	*Guild*	*Hospital*	*Years*	*Sheriff*	*Mayor*
Wylcox, Roger	Cloth-worker	Christ's	1581–86		
Young, Richard	Grocer	St. Bart's	1564–79 & 1580–86		
Young, Robert	Fish-monger	St. Thomas	1564–67		
Young, William	?	St. Bart's	1574–75		

Notes

Preface

1. Ian W. Archer, *The Pursuit of Stability: Social Relations in Elizabethan London* (London: Cambridge University Press, 1991); Paul Slack, *Poverty and Policy in Tudor & Stuart England* (New York: Longman, 1988); Steve Rappaport, *Worlds Within Worlds: Structures of Life in Sixteenth-Century London* (London: Cambridge University Press, 1989); Paul S. Seaver, *Wallington's World: A Puritan Artisan in Seventeenth-Century London* (Stanford, Calif.: Stanford University Press, 1985); A. L. Beier and Roger Finlay, eds., *London 1500–1700: The Making of the Metropolis* (New York: Longman, 1986); Jeremy Boulton, *Neighbourhood and Society: A London Suburb in the Seventeenth Century* (Cambridge: Cambridge University Press, 1987); and Susan Brigden, *London and the Reformation* (New York: Oxford University Press, 1989).

2. John Howes, *Contemporaneous Account, in Dialogue Form of the Foundation and Early History of Christ's Hospital and of Bridewell and St Thomas' Hospitals* (printed from the original manuscript of 1582 & 1587; London, 1889), p. 9. I had the opportunity to compare this printed book with the original manuscript, and it is a good transliteration.

3. For the best use of diaries as evidence on the history of childhood, see Linda A. Pollock's *Forgotten Children: Parent-Child Relations from 1500 to 1900* (New York: Cambridge University Press, 1983) and idem, *A Lasting Relationship: Parents and Children over Three Centuries* (Hanover, N.H.: University Press of New England, 1987). Pollock, in both books, gives a good analysis of the status of the debate over the nature of childhood in the past.

4. See Lloyd De Mause, ed., *The History of Childhood* (London: Souvenir Press, 1976) and Lawrence Stone, *The Family, Sex and Marriage in England 1500–1800* (London: Weidenfeld & Nicolson, 1977).

Introduction: London in 1552

1. Steen Eler Rasmussen, *London: The Unique City*, revised edition (Cambridge, Mass.: Mint Press, 1982), 51.

2. Roger Finlay, *Population and Metropolis: The Demography of London, 1580–1650* (New York: Cambridge University Press, 1981), xi.

3. Harold Priestley, *London: The Years of Change* (London: Frederick Muller, 1966), 29–30.

4. Peter Clark and Paul Slack, *English Towns in Transition* (Toronto: University of Toronto Press, 1972), 64.

5. John Pound, *Poverty and Vagrancy in Tudor England* (London: Longman, 1982).

6. See I. S. W. Blanchard, "Population Change, Enclosure and the Early Tudor Economy," *Economic History Review*, 2d ser., 23, no. 3 (1970): 427–45. J. D. Chambers, *Population, Economy and Society in Pre-Industrial England* (London: Oxford University Press, 1972); J. Cornwall, "English Population in the Early Sixteenth Century," *Economic History Review*, 1970, 32–44; and M. W. Flinn, *The European Demographic System, 1500–1820* (Baltimore: Johns Hopkins University Press, 1981).

7. See J. Thirsk, ed., *Agricultural History of England and Wales*, vol. 4 (Cambridge: Cambridge University Press, 1967).

8. See R. B. Outhwaite, *Inflation in Tudor and Early Stuart England* (London: Macmillan, 1969). "[B]ut at its most rapid, in the middle decades of the sixteenth century, it aroused great concern, especially coming as it did after a century or more of relative price stability. It was also more rapid and sustained than anything experienced in England during the early middle ages or the three centuries following the sixteenth" (p. 9).

9. See Leslie Clarkson, *Death, Disease and Famine in Pre-Industrial England* (New York: St. Martin's Press, 1975); and Paul Slack, "Mortality Crises and Epidemic Disease in England, 1485–1610," in *Health, Medicine and Mortality in the Sixteenth Century*, ed. Charles Webster (Cambridge: Cambridge University Press, 1979).

10. See W. G. Hoskins, "Harvest Fluctuations and the English Economic History, 1480–1619," *Agricultural History Review* 12 (1968).

11. See G. W. O. Woodward, *The Dissolution of the Monasteries* (London: Blanford, 1966).

12. Victor Skipp, *Crisis and Development: An Ecological Study of the Forest of Arden 1570–1674* (Cambridge: Cambridge University Press, 1978), 3.

13. Cornwall, "English Population,"44

14. John Hatcher, *Plague, Population and the English Economy, 1348–1530* (London: Macmillan, 1977), 69. Hatcher claims that by using Gregory King's date, Cornwall overestimated the population eligible for military service.

15. E. A. Wrigley and R. S. Schofield, *The Population History of England, 1541–1871: A Reconstruction* (Cambridge: Harvard University Press, 1981), 208, table 7.8.

16. A. L. Beier and Roger Finlay, *London 1500–1700: The Making of the Metropolis* (London: Longman, 1986), 2.

17. Clark and Slack, *English Towns in Transition*, 83.

18. Ibid.

19. Finlay, *Population and Metropolis*, 51.

20. Peter Clark and Paul Slack, *Crisis and Order in English Towns, 1500–1700* (Toronto: University of Toronto Press, 1972), 35–36.

21. Dunham and Pargellis, *Statutes of the Realm*, 22 Henry VIII, A.D. 1531, 12:423–24.

22. Howes, *Contemporaneous Account, in Dialogue Form of the Foundation and Early History of Christ's Hospital and Bridewell and St. Thomas Hospitals* (printed from the original manuscript of 1582 & 1587; London, 1889), 11.

23. A. L. Beier, "Vagrants and the Social Order in Elizabethan England," *Past and Present* 64 (1974): 15.

24. Quoted from Charles Pendrill, *Old Parish Life in London* (London: Oxford University Press, 1937), 215.

25. "The Citizens of London To The Privy Council on their Suit to the King For Bridewell, 1552," in R. H. Tawney and Eileen Power, eds., *Tudor Economic Documents* (London: Longman, Green, 1951): 306.

26. Howes, *Contemporaneous Account,* 9.

27. Beier, "Vagrants," 4.

28. Ibid., 7–12.

29. D. M. Palliser, *The Age of Elizabeth: England under the Later Tudors, 1547–1603* (New York: Longman, 1983), 129.

30. Howes, *Contemporaneous Account,* 11. Howes's addition is not correct at 2,160.

31. Paul Slack, *Poverty and Policy in Tudor and Stuart England* (New York: Longman, 1988), 24–25.

32. Ibid., 13.

33. William Huse Dunham, Jr., and Stanley Parcellis, eds., *Complaint and Reform in England, 1436–1714* (New York: Oxford University Press, 1938), 423.

34. Henry Arthington, *Provision for the Poore* (London: Thomas Creede, printer, 1597), 4.

35. Slack, *Poverty and Policy,* 26.

36. Edmund Blunden et al., *The Christ's Hospital Book* (London: Hamish Hamilton, 1953), 5–6.

37. Tawney and Power, "Citizens of London," 307.

38. Slack, *Poverty and Policy,* 23.

39. Arthington, *Provision for the Poore,* 2.

40. Slack, *Poverty and Policy,* 22.

41. Ian W. Archer, *The Pursuit of Stability: Social Relations in Elizabethan London* (New York: Cambridge University Press, 1991), 154.

42. David Cressy, *Education in Tudor and Stuart England* (London: Edward Arnold, 1975), 5.

43. Susan Brigden, *London and the Reformation* (New York: Oxford University Press, 1989), 318.

44. Slack, *Poverty and Policy,* 10.

45. J. F. Firth, ed., *Memoranda, References and Documents Relating to the Royal Hospitals of the City of London* (London: Benjamin Pardon, 1803), 80.

46. Philip Gavitt, *Charity and Children in Renaissance Florence: The Ospedale degli Innocenti, 1410–1536* (Ann Arbor: University of Michigan Press, 1990), 107.

Chapter 1. The Solution: The Royal Hospitals

1. The only exception was in the year 1592, when private elections were held because of "the present danger of the infection of the plague. . . ." C.L.R.O., rep. 23.

2. John Howes, *Contemporaneous Account, in Dialogue Form of the Foundation and Early History of Christ's Hospital and of Bridewell and St. Thomas' Hospitals* (printed from the original manuscript of 1582 & 1587; London, 1889), 9. It is unclear whether old age

was in and of itself considered an infirmity or whether it was just observed that older people tend to suffer from more illnesses.

3. Ben Weinreb and Christopher Hibbert, eds., *The London Encyclopaedia* (Bethesda, Md.: Adler & Adler, 1986), 767. "Its name, The Hospital of St. Thomas the Martyr, cannot have been assumed until after Becket's canonization in 1173."

4. Ibid. The Letters Patent establishing the hospitals (26 June 1553) is the first document to record the hospital's change of patron from St. Thomas of Canterbury to St. Thomas the Apostle. E. M. McInnes, *St. Thomas Hospital* (London: George Allen & Unwin, 1963), 24.

5. John Stow, *A Survey of London*, edited by Charles Lethbridge Kingsford from the 1603 edition (1908; reprint, Oxford: Oxford University Press, 1971), 2:144.

6. R. H. Tawney and E. Power, *Tudor Economic Documents* (London: Longmans, Green, 1951), 2:306–8.

7. Stow, *Survey of London*, 2:143.

8. Weinreb and Hibbert, *The London Encyclopaedia*, 86.

9. Howes, *Contemporaneous Account*, 9–10.

10. Guildhall Library manuscript (henceforth, G.L. MS) 12806/1–3, 27 September 1557. Because there are no page numbers, and the folio numbers are often not legible, references will be to date only.

11. Weinreb and Hibbert, *The London Encylopaedia*, 694.

12. Jordan, *Charities of London*, 187.

13. Stow, *Survey of London*, 2:143.

14. E. J. Davies, "The Transformation of London," in *Tudor Studies, Presented to A. F. Pollard*, ed. R. W. Seton-Watson (London: Longman, 1924), 302.

15. Gweneth Whitteridge and Veronica Stokes, *A Brief History of the Hospital of Saint Bartholomew's* (London: Governors of the Hospital of Saint Bartholomew, 1961), 15–17.

16. The City is that part of London contained within the city walls and administered by the corporation; it contained twenty-six wards as of 1603: Portsoken, Tower Street, Aldgate, Limestreet, Bishopsgate, Broad Street, Cornhill, Langbourne, Billingsgate, Bridgeward, Candlewick, Walbrooke, Downgate, Vintry, Cordwainer, Cheap, Coleman Street, Bassishaw, Cripplegate, Aldersgate, Faringdon Within, Breadstreet, Queenhithe, Castle Baynards, Faringdon Without, and the Borough of Southwark and Bridge Ward Without. Unless specifically stated otherwise, reference to London is meant to refer to the City so described, not to metropolitan London.

17. Charles Carlton, *The Court of Orphans* (England: Leicester University Press, 1974), 13. No date is given by Carlton for the establishment of the Court of Orphans as a formal court. He does place the 1530s as a time for reform of the court: see p. 24.

18. Margaret R. Kollock, *The Lord Mayor and Alderman of London during the Tudor Period* (Philadelphia: John C. Winston, 1906), 86.

19. Tawney and Power, *Tudor Economic Documents*, 2:309.

20. Howes, *Contemporaneous Account*, 9.

21. Carlton, *Court of Orphans*, 13.

22. J. F. Firth, ed., *Memoranda, References and Documents Relating to the Royal Hospitals of the City of London* (London: Benjamin Pardon, 1803), 59–60 (26 June, 7 Edward VI, 1553). At the end of this document is the following note: "The foregoing is a true copy of the translation of the Original charter, made by M. Jonathan Hewlett, in February

1809, and examined therewith this 3d day of March 1828, by us, [signed] Thomas Wilby [and] George Trollope[,] Christ's Hospital."

23. See G. W. O. Woodward, *The Dissolution of the Monasteries* (London: Blanford, 1966).

24. See A. G. Dickens, *The English Reformation* (New York: Schocken, 1974).

25. Davies, "Transformation of London," 288.

26. G.L., MS 12806/1, 27 September 1557.

27. Stow, *Survey of London,* 1:318.

28. Howes, *Contemporaneous Account,* 13.

29. Stow, *Survey of London,* 1:319–20

30. Ibid., 322.

31. John Gough Nichols, ed., *Chronicle of the Grey Friars of London* (London: Camden Society, 1852), xx.

32. Stow, *Survey of London,* 1:318.

33. Ibid., 319.

34. Davies, "Transformation of London," 303. The origin of the name of the orphanage is not to be found in the documents. It was probably named after the neighboring Christ Church.

35. Nichols, *Chronicle of the Grey Friars*, xxiii.

36. Sir George Nicholls, *A History of the English Poor Law* (New York: Augustus M. Kelley, 1967), 1:129–34.

37. Firth, *Memoranda, References,* 1.

38. W. K. Jordan, *Edward VI: The Threshold of Power, the Dominance of the Duke of Northumberland* (Cambridge: Harvard University Press, 1970), 219.

39. Howes, *Contemporaneous Account,* 8.

40. Neil L. Kunze, "The Origins of Modern Social Legislation: The Henrician Poor Law of 1536," *Albion* 3 (1971): 10.

41. E. H. Pearce, *Annals of Christ's Hospital* (London: Methuen, 1901), 21. I do not know if this portrait still exists.

42. Howes, *Contemporaneous Account,* 9.

43. Ibid., 11. The total came to 2110. Howes's arithmetic is not correct. He totals the groups and gets 2160.

44. Ibid., 12.

45. Ibid.

46. Ibid.

47. G.L., MS 12819/1–2.

48. Stow, *Survey of London,* 2:25.

49. William Trollope, *A History of the Royal Foundation of Christ's Hospital* (London: William Pickering, 1834), 41.

50. Weinreb and Hibbert, *The London Encyclopaedia,* 743–44.

51. Stow, *Survey of London,* 1:319. The children of Christ's Hospital were called "Bluecoat Boys" because of their distinctive blue coats. It is curious that in their first public appearance they were dressed in red, but they went to blue shortly thereafter.

52. Henry R. Wheatley, *London Past and Present* (London: Singing Tree Press, 1968), 1:394. Originally published in London by John Murraty in 1891.

53. Mark Twain, *The Prince and the Pauper* (New York: New American Library, 1964), 28.

54. Phillis Cunnington and Catherine Lucas, *Charity Costumes of Children, Scholars; Almsfolk, Pensioners* (New York: Harper & Row, 1978), 78–79. Westminster Blue Coat School and York Blue Coat School are but two examples of other schools with a blue coat as part of their uniform.

55. Ibid., 30.

56. Ibid., 77.

57. Ibid.

58. Dr. William Hamilton Fyfe, "The Old Bluecoat School," in *The Barnwell Addresses*, ed. John Louis Haney (Philadelphia: Mary Gaston Barnwell Foundation, 1937), 2:293.

59. Eleanor Farjeon and Herbert Farjeon, *Kings and Queens*, illustrated by Robin Jacques (London: J. M. Dent, 1983), 34.

60. Cunnington and Lucas, *Charity Costumes*, 100–101.

61. John Gough Nichols, ed., *Diary of Henry Machin, 1550–1563*, Camden Society Publication no. 42 (London: Camden Society, 1848), 19 April 1557.

62. G.L., MS 12806/1–2 and Cunnington and Lucas, *Charity Costumes*, 45.

63. G.L., MS 12819/1, June 1555.

64. Trollope, *History of the Royal Foundation*, 41.

65. *A Psalm of Thanksgiving to be Sung by the Children of Christ's Hospital* (London: 1610), quoted from Jordan, *Edward VI*, 192.

Chapter 2. The Structure and Administration

1. J. F. Firth, ed., *Memoranda, References, and Documents Relating to the Royal Hospitals of the City of London* (reprint, London: Benjamin Pardon, 1803), 77.
2. Ibid., 78.
3. Ibid., 84.
4. Ibid., 85.
5. Ibid., 84–85.
6. Ibid., 85.
7. G.L., MS 12806/1, 27 September 1557.
8. Ibid., 15 February 1560/61.
9. Ibid., 19 March, 1560/61.
10. Ibid., vol. 2, 19 July 1572.
11. Ibid., vol. 1, 29 January 1559/60.
12. Firth, *Memoranda, References*, 85.
13. Ibid., 81.
14. Ibid., 85.
15. Ibid.
16. Ibid.
17. See chapter 5 for further information on the presidents and governors.
18. Firth, *Memoranda, References*, 77–78.
19. G.L., MS 12806/1, 1556.
20. Ibid., 1556.
21. Firth, *Memoranda, References*, 78.
22. Ibid.

23. Ibid., 79.
24. Ibid., 78.
25. C.L.R.O., rep.15, fol. 472.
26. Michaelmas is the feast of St. Michael the Archangel. It is also one of the four quarter days; the others are Christmas (25 December); Lady Day (25 March); and Midsummer (24 June).
27. John Stow, *A Survey of London*, ed. Charles Lethbridge Kingsford from the 1603 edition (1908; rpt., Oxford: Oxford University Press, 1971), 2:187.
28. Firth, *Memoranda, References*, 85.
29. Ibid., 78–80.
30. Ibid., 78.
31. Ibid., 79.
32. G.L., MS 12806/1, 2 December 1560.
33. Firth, *Memoranda, References*, 85.
34. Ibid., 85–87.
35. Ibid., 86–87.
36. Ibid., 86.
37. Ibid., 87.
38. G.L., MS 12806/2, 5 April 1560.
39. Firth, *Memoranda, References*, 88.
40. Ibid.
41. Ibid.
42. Ibid.
43. Ibid., 89.
44. Ibid.
45. Ibid.
46. Ibid., 90.
47. Ibid.
48. Ibid., 98.
49. John Howes, *Contemporaneous Account, in Dialogue-Form of the Foundation and Early History of Christ's Hospital and of Bridewell and St. Thomas' Hospitals* (printed from the original manuscript of 1582 & 1587; London, 1889), 15.
50. Ibid.
51. Ibid.
52. Edmund Blunden et al. *The Christ's Hospital Book* (London: Hamish Hamilton, 1953), 7.
53. Howes, *Contemporaneous Account*, 15.
54. Ibid.
54. Ibid.
55. Ibid.
56. Firth, *Memoranda, References*, 92.
57. Ibid.
58. Ibid.
59. Ibid.
60. Ibid.
61. Ibid.
62. Ibid., 93.

63. Ibid.
64. Ibid., 93–94.
65. Ibid., 91–92.
66. Howes, *Contemporaneous Account,* 15.
67. Firth, *Memoranda, References,* 94.
68. Ibid.
69. Ibid.
70. Ibid., 95.
71. Ibid.
72. Ibid., 94.
73. Ibid.
74. Ibid., 95.
75. Ibid., 94–95.
76. G.L., MS 12806/3, 10 November 1593.
77. Ibid., 19 February 1593/1594. The new year started on March 26 according to the Tudor calendar, so that 19 February 1593 was really A.D. 1594.
78. Ibid., 6 July 1594.
79. Ibid., 14 September 1594. A portion was a child's inheritance that was turned over to the hospital for safekeeping until the child reached the age of maturity, most commonly at the age of twenty-one.
80. Ibid., 28 September 1594.
81. Ibid., vol. 2, undated court meeting between 9 December 1570 and 29 January 1570/71.
82. Firth, *Memoranda, References,* 95.
83. Ibid., 96.
84. Ibid., 95.
85. Ibid.
86. Ibid.
87. Ibid., 96.
88. Ibid.
89. Ibid.
90. Ibid.
91. Ibid., 97–98.
92. Ibid., 98.
93. Ibid., 97-98.
94. Ibid., 98.
95. Ibid.
96. Ibid.
97. G.L., MS 12806/l, 4 December 1560.
98. Ibid., 21 October 1560.
99. Firth, *Memoranda, References,* 99.
100. Ibid.
101. Ibid.
102. Ibid.
103. Ibid., 98–99.
104. Ibid., 99
105. Ibid., 100.

106. Ibid., 79.
107. G.L., MS 12806/3, 22 January 1592/93.
108. Firth, *Memoranda, References,* 97.
109. Ibid.
110. Ibid.
111. Ibid.
112. Ibid., 98.
113. G.L., MS 12806/3, 10 November 1593.
114. Ibid., 14 November 1593.
115. Firth, *Memoranda, References,* 82.
116. G.L., MS 12806/2, 22 July 1592.
117. See the dozens of examples of leases recorded in The Minutes of the Court of Governors.
118. G.L., MS 12806/1, 14 April 1562.
119. Firth, *Memoranda, References,* 82.
120. G.L., MS 12806/2, 24 November 1561.
121. Ibid., 6 May 1570.
122. Ibid., 9 September 1570.
123. Firth, *Memoranda, References,* 84.
124. G.L., MS 12806/2, 19 November 1569.
125. Ibid., 27 November 1569.
126. Ibid.
127. Ibid., 10 December 1569.
128. Ibid., 12 August 1570.
129. Ibid., 14 October 1570.
130. Ibid., 9 December 571.
131. Jack Goody, *The Development of the Family and Marriage in Europe* (New York: Cambridge University Press, 1983), 146–51.
132. G.L., MS 12806/2, undated court meeting sometime between 29 December 1571 and 9 February 1571/72.
133. Ibid., 17 February 1570/71.
134. Ibid., vol. 1, 7 December 1556.
135. Ibid., 14 August 1557.
136. Ibid., vol. 2, 12 March 1568/69.

Chapter 3. Revenues and Sources of Income

1. G.L., MS 12806/2, 31 January 1591/92.
2. During the fiscal year of 1594–95, the treasurer recorded receipts totaling £2883 11s. 11d. 1/2. The entry for that year's account is concluded by the following declaration: "audited by us the Governors of the four hospitals, whose names are hereunto, subscribed, and we do find by this account . . . Master Robert Cogan Treasurer of Christ's Hospital hath disbursed and laid out of his own purse, the sum of fourteen pounds, six shillings, five pence three farthings—as appeareth in the account aforesaid. . . ." The signatures of William Cobb (governor of Bridewell), Robert Campbell (governor of St. Thomas),

Robert Hawes (governor of Christ's), and William Thwaytes (governor of Christ's) are affixed under this audit statement.

3. G.L., MS 12819/1, 1 July 1554–30 June 1555.

4. Ibid., vol. 2, 1 October 1564–30 September 1565.

5. This author has been employed by two nonprofit organizations within the last five years, and it is truly amazing how many things people will donate in lieu of a cash donation, even though money can be an income tax deduction. Some people seem to regard charities as a convenient place to dump unwanted items and do not seem to consider that maybe their donation is unwanted because it is junk.

6. G.L., MS 12819/1, 1553.

7. Ibid., 23 November 1555. Watchet is defined as "A light blue colour; cloth or garments of this colour." *Oxford Universal English Dictionary*, s.v. "watchet."

8. G.L., MS 12,819/2, 29 September 1582–29 September 1583.

9. G.L., MS 12,806/2, 30 November–17 January 1563/64. The extant parish records during this time are fragmentary, which makes it difficult, if not impossible, to reconstruct collections from the vantage point of the parishes themselves.

10. Roger Finlay, *Population and Metropolis: The Demography of London, 1580–1800* (New York: Cambridge University Press, 1981), 168–71.

11. G.L., MS 12,806/2, 18 March 1591/92.

12. Ibid., 29 September 1596–29 September 1597.

13. Ibid., 29 September 1593-29 September 1594.

14. C.L.R.O., jour. 21, fol. 230.

15. G.L., MS 12819/1, 13 April 1557.

16. William Kent, ed., *An Encyclopaedia of London* (London: J. M.Dent, 1970). When Tudor Londoners talked about foreigners, they were talking about anyone, including other Englishmen, who lived outside of London. Sometimes, "foreigner" could also refer to anyone outside of one's parish.

17. G.L. MS. 12806/3, 22 January 1594/95.

18. Ibid., vol. 2, 29 September 1581–29 September 1582.

19. Ibid., 29 September 1597–29 September 1598.

20. Ibid., 29 September 1587–29 September 1588.

21. Ibid., 29 September 1579–29 September 1580. In Tudor usage the term *tenement* did not mean slum, which is now the common meaning of this word. A tenement was simply a piece of real estate.

22. Ibid., 29 September 1582–29 September 1583.

23. Ibid., 29 September 1576–29 September 1577.

24. Ibid., 19 September 1590–29 September 1591.

25. Ibid., 29 September 1597–29 September 1598.

26. Ibid.

27. Ibid., 29 September 1581–29 September 1582.

28. Ibid., 29 September 1597–29 September 1598.

29. *Oxford English Dictionary*, s.v. "legacy."

30. G.L., MS 12819/1, 18 May 1555.

31. W. K. Jordan, *The Charities of London, 1480–1660: The Aspirations and the Achievements of the Urban Society* (New York: Russell Sage Foundation, 1960), 28.

32. G.L., 12805/1, 1586.

33. Ibid., 1554–83.

34. Ibid., 1598.

35. Ibid., 1597.

36. George A.T. Allan, ed., *Christ's Hospital Admissions*, vol. 1, *1554–1599* (London: Harrison and Sons, 1937), 38.

37. Edmund Blunden et al., *The Christ's Hospital Book* (London: Hamish Hamilton, 1953), 10–11.

38. G.L., MS 12,806/3, 13 March 1595/96.

39. George Unwin, *The Guilds and Companies of London* (New York: Barnes & Noble, 1966), 1:356.

40. G.L., MS 12829, 7 May 1582.

41. Phillis Cunnington and Catherine Lucas, *Charity Costumes of Children, Scholars; Almsfolk, Pensioners* (New York: Barnes & Noble, 1978), 52.

42. G.L., MS 12819/2, 29 September 1587–29 September 1588.

43. Ibid.

44. C.L.R.O., rep., fol. 311.

45. G. L. MS. 3339 (Box A) "the Prosedinge at the funeral of Skynner esquier who died Lo. Maiore of London & was buryed as a barron."

46. *O.E.D.*, s.v. "worsted wool."

47. G.L., MS 12,819/2, 29 September 1587–29 September 1588.

48. Bay is defined as "A reddish brown colour; used esp. of horses." *O.E.D.*, s.v. "bay."

49. Lotus 1-2-3, the program used to generate the graphs for this book, only allows eight parts to a pie chart. Since Christ's Hospital had eleven major sources of income, this forced the lumping of the four least bountiful sources (benevolence, annuities, boxes, and Bay Hall) into a miscellaneous category.

50. *O.E.D.*, s.v. "benevolence."

51. G.L., MS 12819/2, 1 October 1562–30 September 1563.

52. Ibid., 29 September 1579–29 September 1580.

53. Ibid., vol. 1, 1554.

54. Ibid., vol. 2, 1 October 1562–30 September 1563.

55. Ibid., 29 September 1576–29 September 1577.

56. Ibid., 29 September 1579–29 September 1580.

57. Ibid., 1 October 1563–30 September 1564.

58. Ibid., 1 October 1562–30 September 1563.

59. Ibid., 29 September 1582–29 September 1583.

60. Ibid. This is probably Richard Gurney, who served as a sheriff in 1589 and served as a governor of Christ's Hospital from 1588 to 1596.

61. Ibid., vol. 1, 26 August 1555.

62. Ibid., vol. 2, 20 September 1571–20 September 1572.

63. Allan, *Christ's Hospital Admissions,* 105.

64. G.L., MS 12819/2, 29 September 1589–29 September 1590.

65. Ibid., 20 September 1570–20 September 1571.

66. Ibid., 20 September 1571–20 September 1572.

67. Ibid., 29 September 1575–29 September 1576.

68. Ibid., 1 October 1565–30 September 1566.

69. C.F.R.O., rep. 16, fol. 454.

70. G.L., MS 12819/1, 7 May 1555.
71. Ibid., 23 November 1555.
72. Ibid., 29 September 1597–29 September 1598.
73. Ibid., 29 September 1581–29 September 1582.
74. Ibid., 29 September 1574–29 September 1575.
75. A wardmote is "A meeting of the citizens of a ward; esp. in the City of London, a meeting of the liverymen of a ward under the presidency of the alderman." In other words, it is "a judicial inquiry made by a ward. . . ." *O.E.D.*, s.v. "wardmote."
76. G.L., MS 4069/1, fols. 42–82.
77. G.L., 12819/1, p. 70.
78. Ibid., vol. 2, 1 October 1561–30 September 1562.
79. Ibid., 29 September 1597–29 September 1598.
80. See Peter H. Ramsey, ed., *The Price Revolution in Sixteenth-Century England* (London: Methuen, 1971); C. J. Harrison,"Grain Price Analysis and Harvest Qualities, 1465-1634," *Agricultural History Review* 19 (1971); E. H. Phelps Brown and Sheila V. Hopkins, "Seven Centuries of the Prices of Consumables, compared with Builders' Wage-rates," *Economica*, n.s. 203, no. 92 (1956); J. Thirsk, ed., *The Agrarian History of England and Wales*, vol. 4, *1500–1640* (Cambridge: Cambridge University Press, 1967).
81. G.L., MS 12806/2, 18 December 1591.
82. Ibid., 1 December 1591.
83. Ibid., vol. 3, July 1595.
84. Ibid.
85. Ibid., 14 February 1597/98.
86. Ibid., vol. 2, 21 September 1590.
87. Ibid., vol. 3, 24 March 1594/95.
88. Ibid., 10 September 1595.
89. Ibid., 19 May 1598.
90. Peter J. Bowden, *The Wool Trade in Tudor and Stuart England*, rev. ed. (London: Frank Cass, 1971), appendix. This was originally published in 1962 by St. Martin's Press.
91. G.L., MS 12806/2, undated document at the end of the volume.
92. Ibid., undated document at the end of the volume with the title of "the Scrutenars charge / which is to be read and declared at his receiving in to the house in presence of the courts."
93. Ibid., vol. 1, 19 November 1560.
94. Ibid.
95. Ibid., vol. 3, 4 November 1592.
96. Ibid.
97. Ibid., 21 September 1596. Wheat prices that year were the highest of the century.
98. Ibid., 6 March 1957/98.

Chapter 4. Expenditures: The Cost of Running Christ's Hospital

1. This is not unexpected; labor costs are consistently the most expensive part of most modern institutional budgets.

2. G.L., MS. 12819/1–2. The treasurer's accounts are missing for 1560 and are incomplete for 1561 and 1593. This causes some statistical abnormalities in the graphs.

3. Ibid., vol. 1, 15 April 1553.

4. Ibid., 22 April, 1553.

5. Ibid., vol. 2, 29 September 1582–29 September 1583.

6. Staff expenditures included: beadle, board wages, clerk, clerk/overseer, coalhouse keeper, dublet, fees, livery, livery/nurse&mat, matron, matron/diet, matron/livery, matron/nurses, matron's dietmaid, morgan, morgan/diet, officer/c.h., officer/c.h.&stt, officers/c.h., porter, sexton/x'schurch, staff, stafftorch usher, wage/diet, wages, wages/fees, waterbearer. (See Appendix A.)

7. G.L., MS 12819/1, June 1553.

8. Ibid., July 1554

9. Ibid., vol. 2, 29 September 1597–29 September 1598.

10. Acates (miscellaneous food), acates/milk, ale, apple pies, barrel butter, baysalt, beef/mutton, beer, beer/bread, beer/carriage, bread, butter, butter/carriage, butter/cheese, carrotroot, carrots/pepper, cheese, cheese/carriage (transportation cost), Dutch fish, Dutch herring, Essex butter, Essex cheese, great oatmeal, grocer, herbes, herring, herring/carriage, herring/fish, herring/spratt, honey, mackerel/carriage, meat, milk, misc/acates, misc/food, mutton, newland cod (fish caught off the coast of Newfoundland), newland fish/carriage, oatmeal, pepper, playse, playse/carriage, playse/fish, provisions, raisins, red herring, red spratt, salt, salt/carriage, salt butter, Sotherie butter, spratt, Suffolk butter, Suffolk cheese, Surrey butter, sweet butter, vinegar, week's diet, wheat, white/wheat bread, white bread, white salt, white salt/baysalt, white salt/carriage, whyting, whyting/carriage, yeast, yeast/herbes. (See Appendix A.)

11. See Jack C. Drummond and Anne Wilbraham, *The Englishman's Food: A History of Five Centuries of English Diet* (London: Jonathan Cape, 1939). For a further discussion of the role of food and drink not solely for Europeans but also for the rest of the world, see Fernand Braudel, *Capitalism and Material Life, 1400–1800* (New York: Harper & Row, 1967), chaps. 2 and 3.

12. G.L., MS 12806/1, 8 November 1557.

13. G.L., MS 12819/1, 1 June 1555.

14. G.L., MS 12806/2, March 20 1591/1592.

15. Ibid., vol. 3, 7 April 1595.

16. G.L. MS 12819/1, 17 August 1555.

17. Bartholomew of England, *De proprietatibus rerum*, lib. 6, *De proprietatibus aetatum* (Frankfurt, 1601), 241. Quoted from Mary Martin McLaughlin, "Survivors and Surrogates," in *The History of Childhood*, ed. Lloyd de Mause (New York: Harper & Row, 1974), 115.

18. James Bruce Ross, "The Middle-Class Child in Urban Italy," in de Mause, *The History of Childhood*, 187.

19. Palolo da Certaldo, *Libro di buoni costumi*, in Donato Velluti, *La cronica domestica (1367–1370)*, ed. I. del Lungo and G. Volpi (Florence, 1914); and Giovanni di Pagolo Morelli, *Ricordi*, 2d ed., ed. Vittore Branca (Florence, 1969), 234, quoted from James Bruce Ross "The Middle-Class Child in Urban Italy," in de Mause, *The History of Childhood*, 187.

20. The following varieties of fish were listed: playse, which is a kind of flounder; different varities of herring; Newfoundland fish, which is probably cod; mackerel, sprat, which is a small herring, and whiting.

21. E. H. Pearce, *Annals of Christ's Hospital* (London: Methuen, 1901), 176.

22. Charles Dickens, *Oliver Twist* (New York: Bantam Books, 1982), 12–13.

23. "The Order of the Hospitalls of K. Henry the viijth and K. Edward the vith, viz. St. Bartholomew's Christ's, Bridewell, St. Thomas's by the Maior, Cominaltie, and Citizens of London, Governours of the Possessions, Revenues, and Goods of the sayd hospitalls" in *Memoranda, References, and Documents Relating to the Royal Hospitals of the City of London,* ed. J. K. Firth (rpt., London: Benjamin Pardon, 1803), 87.

24. G.L. MS 12806/1, 15 July 1560.

25. Ibid., 30 January 1558/59

26. Ibid., 11 March 1559/60.

27. Ibid., 21 October 1560.

28. Ibid., 29 April 1560.

29. Ibid., 19 November 1560.

30. Ibid.

31. Ibid., 20 January 1560/1561.

32. Ibid., 2 July 1561.

33. Ibid., 26 March 1561/62.

34. Ibid., 24 November 1561.

35. Ibid.

36. G.L., MS 12819/2, 6 July 1594.

37. Ibid., 1552–57

38. Apron, Baie/white cotton, baie cloth, baies, bay's white, black cap, black cotton, black freise, black lace, black thread, blanket, blue cloth, bluecloth/dressing, blue kersey, broad blue cloth, broad white cloth, brown canvas, caddas, calve skin, canvas, canvas/greenclot, canvas/holland, canvas/lockeram, cloth, cloth/dressing, cloth/misc, cloth and dressing, clothing, clothworking, coarse inckle, coat, cotton, corked shoe, dowlas, dressing, dressing/trimmin, dutch white canvas, dying, dying ofy arn, fell wool, fine cloth/dressing, fine dowlas, fine green cloth, fine inckle, flax, fleece wool, forfeit leather, freise, fuling, fulling/cloth, fulling/wool, gents holland, green cloth, green cuslens, green wadmoll, greenwood mallin, harford, hides, holland cloth, holland hemp, holland linen, hosen, hosen/mending, hosen/shoes, kersies, knit hosen, lace, laste/shoes, leather, leather/carriage, leather/dressing, leather girdle, leather points, linen, linen/greencloth, linen yarn, lockeram, lynsis wolsey, manchester freise, misc/clothing, n.cloth/dressing, n.gray/ dressing, n.kersy/dressing, n.straight/dress, narrow baie, night cappes, normand canvas, northern cloth, northern gray, northern paline, northern russet, north straigh, petticoat, plain/ greycloth, plainwhite, redlace, roan canvas, rough flax, russet petticoat, sewing thread, shoes, shoes/mend petico, shorflax, shrink/wet, smock, sole leather, solte wyche, coultege, straw hats, suffolk/dressing, suffolk blue cloth, thread, weaving, weaving/linen, weaving/napkin, weaving/wool, weaving/yarn, welch baies, welch cotton, welch freise, wet/set, white baie/cotton, white baies, white canvas, white cloth, white cotton, white gloucesters, white grasier, white hartford, white herford, white owedplain, white welch cotton, white welsh baie, white ynckle, woolen card, woolen yarn, woolen yarn/hosen, yarn, ynckle comb. (See Appendix A.)

39. G.L., MS 12819/2, 20 September 1566–20 September 1567.

40. Ibid., 20 September 1566–20 September 1567.

41. William H. Te Brake, "Air Pollution and Fuel Crises in Preindustrial London, 1250–1650," *Technology & Culture* 16 (1975): 337.

42. The category of candles is aggregated out of items that were not exclusively candles, but all bear some relationship to providing light. Because candles were the main purchase in this category, I will refer to the following entries as simply candles: candle/wick, candles, candlestick, cotton candles, glass lantern, lamp oil, moskova [Moscow] tallow, oil for lamp/soap, tallow, tallow/carriage, watching candle, whale oil, wick candle.

43. G.L., MS 12819/2, 27 September 1567.

44. Sir Lesley Stephen and Sir Sidney Lee, eds., *Dictionary of National Biography* (London: Oxford University Press, 1949–50), 4:204–5.

45. G.L., MS 12819/2, 29 September 1596–29 September 1597.

46. Ibid., 29 September 1589–29 September 1590.

47. Ibid., vol. 1, April 1553.

48. Ibid., vol. 2, 29 September 1582–29 September 1583.

49. Ibid. I assume the reference here is to the solicitor-general, Sir Thomas Egerton, who served in that office from 1581 to 1591. See Arthur F. Kinney, *Titled Elizabethans: A Directory of Elizabethan State and Church Officers and Knights, with Peers of England, Scotland, and Ireland, 1558–1603* (Hamden, Conn.: Archon Books, 1973), 7.

50. Ibid., 29 September 1595–29 September 1596. The hospital's treasurer at this date was Robert Cogan. The Court of Aldermen had determined in 1576 that if any officers of any of the hospitals were "beaten or misused by any person," then that person would be punished as determined by two of the aldermen, one of whom had to be a justice of the peace [C.L.R.O., rep. 19, fol. 89].

51. Ibid., 29 September 1583–29 September 1584.

52. Ibid. I have not tabulated this £1 in with other legal expenses due to its special nature.

53. Lawrence Stone, *The Crisis of the Aristocracy, 1558–1641,* abridged edition (London: Oxford University Press, 1967), 118.

54. G.L., MS 12819/1, December 1553.

55. Ibid., 14 April 1554.

56. Ibid., April 1553.

57. Ibid., 5 October 1555.

58. Ibid., 8 April 1553.

59. Ibid., March 1554.

60. Ibid., vol. 2, 29 September 1597–29 September 1598.

61. Ibid., vol. 1, May 1553.

62. Ibid., vol. 2, 29 September 1574–29 September 1575.

63. Ibid., 29 September 1585–29 September 1586.

64. Ibid., 29 September 1580–29 September 1581.

65. Ibid., vol. 1, 28 February 1555/56.

66. Ibid., vol. 2, 1 October 1562–30 September 1563.

67. Ibid., 1 October 1563–30 September 1564.

68. Ibid., 29 September 1576–29 September 1577.

69. Ibid., 29 September 1577–29 September 1578.

70. Ibid., 29 September 1596–29 September 1597. Good plumbing was required for the wash house, which was probably used in large measure for the processing and preparing of cloth and not just for cleaning dirty linen and other laundry.

71. Ibid., 1 October 1563–30 September 1564.

72. Ibid., 1 October 1565–30 September 1566.

73. Ibid., 20 September 1571–20 September 1572. In 1575, a sum of £45 13s. 2d. was invested in "Repracions upon the old sick ward for Mr Waddington's house," which leads to the assumption that the old sick ward was turned into a lodging.

74. Ibid., 29 September 1576–29 September 1577. The Counting House was probably where the treasurers and clerks worked and where the hospital's money was kept.

75. Ibid., 29 September 1580–29 September 1581.

76. John Gough Nichols, ed., *The Diary of Henry Machin, Citizen and Merchant-Taylor of London from A.D. 1550 to A.D. 1563,* Camden Society Publication no. 42 (London: Camden Society, 1848), 3. This would appear to be the day after Easter. Easter seems to have fallen on 18 April in that year. See C. R. Cheney, ed., *Handbook of Dates for Students of English History* (London: Royal Historical Society, 1945), 159.

77. G.L., MS 12819/2, 29 September 1589–29 September 1590.

78. Ibid., 29 September 1595–29 September 1596.

79. Ibid.

80. Ibid., 29 September 1593–29 September 1594.

81. Ibid., 29 September 1594–29 September 1595.

82. G.L., MS 12806/3, 21 February 1595/96.

83. G.L., MS 12819/1, 29 September 1594-29 September 1595.

84. Ibid., vol. 2, 29 September 1594-29 September 1595.

85. Ibid., 29 September 1583-29 September 1584.

86. Ibid., vol. 1, May 1553.

87. Ibid., April 1553.

88. Ibid., vol. 2, 1 October 1564–30 September 1565.

89. Ibid., 5 February 1585/86.

90. Ibid., 29 September 1582–29 September 1583.

91. Ibid., 29 September 1591–29 September 1592.

92. Ibid., 29 September 1584–29 September 1585.

93. Ibid., 29 September 1582–29 September 1583.

94. Ibid., 29 September 1587–29 September 1588.

95. Ibid., 29 September 1596–29 September 1597.

96. Ibid., vol. 1, December 1553.

97. Ibid., vol. 2, 29 September 1581–29 September 1582.

98. For example, the £404 11s. 11d. debited to the Blackwell Hall account in the fiscal year of 1595–96 is broken down in the following manner: "Payments Out Blackwell Hall" £200 paid to the treasurer of St. Bartholomew's Hospital "towards the relief of the poor there, for a year. . . ." This annual payment of £200 is not included in the debits for Blackwell Hall by me, because it makes more sense to put it in with the account for the other hospitals. The sum of £33 6s. 8d. was additionally paid to the treasurer of St. Barts "for rent of Blackwell Hall. . . ." Five pounds was given "To the Chamber of London for the Library. . . ." A total of £12 13s. 4d. was paid out "for rent of the Room." The amount of £1 6s. 8d. was spent "for rent of the Gallery near Guildhall chapel. . . ." One shilling was dispensed "for rent of the Town Ditch. . . ." "Paid to Officers of the same hall." Thirty-five pounds was salaried "to George Newbolds keeper of Blackwell Hall." Twenty pounds was paid "To William Hawleie clerk of the Storehouse. . . ." Ten pounds was the annual salary of each of the eight clerks: Thomas Leedame, Robert Seacole, Oliver Goddarde, Henry Colsone, Edward Glouer, Thomas Martine, Morgan

Llewellen, and Oliver Jones. Five pounds was half a year's salary paid to Thomas Bowyer. Five pounds each was annually paid to William Gibson and Robert Androwes. A total of £3 15s. was paid "To Lewis Jenkynnes for 3/4 of a yeere. . . ." The sum of £2 13s. 4d. was discharged "To the Parson of Michaell Bassieshawe for Tithe" The sum of £1 13s. was dispensed "To the scavengers of the same parish. . . ." The amount of £1 8s. 3d. was paid "To the Parsoneof St. Lawrence in the Jury for Tithe. . . ." Three pounds was paid "for, 5, fifteenths granted this year. . . ." A total of 14s. 8d. was the outlay for simply "wages, one year. . . ."

99. G.L., MS 12819/2, 29 September 1589–29 September 1590.

100. Ibid., 1 October 1565–30 September 1566.

101. For example, in the fiscal year of 1595–96, these payments, totaling £63 3s., were dispersed in the following manner: £20 was salaried "To Thomas Swift clerk of the said hall for a year," £42 was allotted "To Mr Connye for rent for the same hall a year," 8s. was given " To the Parson of St Olives in the Jury for tithe," and 15s. was "for fifteenths 4 & 1/2 granted this year. . . ."

102. G.L., MS 12819/1, May 1553.

103. Ibid., vol. 2, 29 September 1582–29 September 1583. The Thames functioned as London's major road, and it was always more efficient to travel by water in Tudor England.

104. Ibid., vol. 1, December, 1553.

105. Ibid.

106. Ibid.

107. Ibid.

108. Ibid., January 1553/54.

109. Ibid., 5 October 1555.

110. Ibid., 12 October 1555.

111. Ibid., 26 November 1555.

112. Ibid., 16 November 1555.

113. Ibid., 30 November 1555. This cross must have been made out of wood, for John Bonde was a carpenter by trade and "stuff" was the common expression to describe materials used in the making of the cross.

114. Ibid., 7 December 1555.

115. Ibid.

116. Ibid., 20 June 1556.

117. Ibid., April 1553.

118. Ibid.

119. Ibid., vol. 2, 29 September 1596–29 September 1597.

120. John Howes, *Contemporaneous Account, in Dialogue Form of the Foundation and Early History of Christ's Hospital and of Bridewell and St. Thomas' Hospitals* (printed from the original manuscript of 1582 & 1587; London: 1889), 43.

121. Mark Twain, *The Prince and the Pauper* (New York: New American Library, 1980), 202.

Chapter 5. Governors and Guardians

1. G.L., MS 12806/2, at the end of the volume, undated.
2. Ibid., undated.

3. Frank Freeman Foster, *The Politics of Stability: A Portrait of the Rulers in Elizabethan London* (London: Royal Historical Society, 1977), 60.

4. G.L., MS 12806/1, 5 April 1560.

5. Ibid.

6. Margaret R. Kollock, *The Lord Mayor and Aldermen of London during the Tudor Period* (Philadelphia: John C. Winston, 1906), 21–22.

7. Foster, *Politics of Stability*, app. 1.

8. This is not to say that these men only served Christ's Hospital in governorships; in fact, most of them also served the other three hospitals as governors. However, I counted any service to Christ's Hospital as a governor, even if it was only for a short period of time.

9. G.L., MS 12806/1–3.

10. Foster, *Politics of Stability*, 63.

11. E. H. Pearce, *Annals of Christ's Hospital* (London: Methuen, 1901), 21.

12. A. B. Beaven, *The Aldermen of the City of London (1908–13)* (London: E. Fisher and Co., 1908–13), 2:33 n. 44.

13. Kollock, *The Lord Mayor*, 67–68.

14. G. D. Ramsay, *The City of London in International Politics at the Accession of Elizabeth Tudor* (Manchester: Manchester University Press, 1975), 35.

15. Ibid., 34–36.

16. Beaven, *Aldermen of London*, 2:33.

17. Ibid., 37.

18. Ibid., 39.

19. Ibid., 40.

20. Foster, *Politics of Stability*, 61.

21. Beaven, *Aldermen of London*, 2:33–40.

22. Kollock, *The Lord Mayor*, 26.

23. Ibid., 23–24.

24. Ibid., 24.

25. Ibid., 64.

26. Ibid., 35.

27. Ibid., 51.

28. Ibid., 17.

29. Ibid., 40–41.

30. Ibid., 62.

31. Ibid., 53.

32. Beaven, *Aldermen of London*, 2:33–39.

33. Sir Leslie Stephen and Sir Sidney Lee, eds., *Dictionary of National Biography* (London: Oxford University Press, 1949–50), 12:176.

34. Kollock, *The Lord Mayor*, 17–19.

35. Beaven, *Aldermen of London*, 2:33.

36. Ibid., 39.

37. Ibid., 39–40.

38. D. M. Palliser, *The Age of Elizabeth: England under the Later Tudors, 1547–1603* (London: Longman, 1983), 216.

39. Stephen and Lee, *Dictionary of National Biography*, 14:899.

40. Ibid., 5:1027.

41. Ramsay, *The City of London,* 360.
42. Beaven, *Aldermen of London,* 2:39.
43. Stephen and Lee, *Dictionary of National Biography,* 14:899.
44. Ibid., 14:900.
45. H. B. Wheatley, ed., *Stow's Survey of London* (New York: Dutton, 1970), 104.
46. G.L., MS. 12812/1, (1552–1820), 1582.
47. Beaven, *Aldermen of London,* 2:37.
48. Ibid., 1:173.
49. Book of Legacies, 1590.
50. Beaven, *Aldermen of London,* 2:39.
51. Stephen and Lee, *Dictionary of National Biography,* 5:1027.
52. John Gough Nichols, ed., *Diary of Henry Machin, 1550–1563,* Camden Society Publication no. 42 (London: Camden Society, 1848), 381nn.
53. Stephen and Lee, *Dictionary of National Biography,* 5:1028.
54. G.L., MS 12806/3, 15 January 1593/94.
55. Pearce, *Annals,* 302. Appendix A.
56. Stephen and Lee, *Dictionary of National Biography,* 12:1176.
57. Ibid.
58. Ibid.
59. G.L., MS 12819/1–2 and C.L.R.O., rep. 13–24.
60. Foster, *Politics of Stability,* 61.
61. Stephen and Lee, *Dictionary of National Biography,* 5:310–12.
62. Ibid., 5:311.
63. Ibid., 5:310.
64. G.L., MS 12819/2, 1 October 1561–30 September 1562.
65. Stephen and Lee, *Dictionary of National Biography,* 5:311.
66. Ibid., 5:312.
67. G.L., MS 12806/2, 1 October 1565–30 September 1566; 20 September 1567–20 September 1568.
68. C.L.R.O., rep. 17, fols. 242 and 312.
69. Stephen and Lee, *Dictionary of National Biography,* 5:310–12.
70. Foster, *Politics of Stability,* 165.
71. G.L., MS 12806/1, 27 September 1559.
72. Ibid., vol. 2, 22 September 1561.
73. Ibid., 30 October 1573.
74. G.L., MS 12812/1, 1582.
75. Ibid., 1593.
76. G.L., MS 12819/2, 29 September 1595–29 September 1596.
77. G.L., MS 12806/1–3 and MS 12819/1–2.
78. Wheatley, *Stow's Survey,* 104.
79. C.L.R.O., rep., 14, fols. 216–17.
80. Howes, *A Contemporaneous Account, in Dialogue Form of the Foundation and Early History of Christ's Hospital and of Bridewell and St. Thomas' Hospitals* (printed from the original manuscript of 1582 & 1587; London, 1889), 48.
81. G.L., MS 12806/2, 21 September 1585.
82. Stephen and Lee, *Dictionary of National Biography,* 5:1028.
83. Ibid., 12:1176.

84. W. K. Jordan, *The Charities of London, 1480–1660: The Aspirations and the Achievements of the Urban Society* (New York: Russell Sage Foundation, 1960), 103–4.

85. Stephen and Lee, *Dictionary of National Biography,* 8:1312.

86. Ibid., 8:1312–13.

87. G.L., MS12819/2, 29 September 1583–29 September 1584.

88. Ibid., 29 September 1586–29 September 1587.

89. G.L., MS12806/2, 31 January 1591/92.

Chapter 6. The Children

1. A detailed statistical study of the children of Christ's Hospital is being undertaken to determine such information as death rates, gender ratios, average age of children, etc.

2. John Gough Nichols, ed., *Literary Remains of King Edward the Sixth* (New York: Burt Franklin, 1964?), 1:clxxxiv.

3. G.L., MS 12818/1, 5 June 1563.

4. G.L., MS 12806/1, 1556.

5. Ian W. Archer, *The Pursuit of Stability: Social Relations in Elizabethan London* (New York: Cambridge University Press, 1991), 157.

6. Ibid.

7. J.F. Firth, ed., *Memoranda, References, and Documents Relating to the Royal Hospitals of the City of London* (London: Benjamin Pardon, 1803), 83.

8. Edmund Blunden et al., *The Christ's Hospital Book* (London: Hamish Hamilton, 1953), 7.

9. G.L., MS 12806/3, 7 April 1593.

10. George A. T. Allan, *Christ's Hospital Admissions*, vol. 1, *1554–1599* (London: Harrison and Sons, 1937), 103 (23 February 1571/72). This is the transliteration of the original Children's Register; I have verified that it is accurate.

11. Ibid., 136 (14 April 1576).

12. Ibid., 83 (10 July 1568).

13. Ibid., 2 (4 October 1557).

14. Ibid., 113 (20 June 1573).

15. Archer, *The Pursuit of Stability,* 157.

16. G.L., MS 12806/2, 28 March 1573.

17. Ibid., vol. 2, 14 November 1565.

18. Allan, *Christ's Hospital Admissions,* 116 (10 October 1573).

19. Ibid., 103 (23 February 1571/72). Also see the entry in G.L., MS 12806/2, 23 February 1571/72.

20. Allan, *Christ's Hospital Admissions,* 158 (10 September 1580).

21. Ibid., 67 (20 October 1565).

22. Ibid., 74 (30 November 1566).

23. G.L., MS 12806/2, 4 October 1570. Philip Gavitt notes the same phenomenon in *Charity and Children in Renaissance Florence: The Ospedale degli Innocenti, 1410–1536* (Ann Arbor: University of Michigan Press, 1990), 188 : "If a parent was diffident, he or she might leave a countersign to identify the child in the event of reclamation. This countersign might be an object, or a drawing on the note pinned to the child's clothing."

24. G.L., MS 12806/2, 28 March 1573.
25. Allan, *Christ's Hospital Admissions,* 9 (16 October 1559).
26. Ibid., 40 (10 April 1563).
27. Ibid., 59 (10 June 1564).
28. Ibid., 52 (6 November 1563)..
29. Ibid., 23 (23 March 1561/62).
30. Ibid., 13 (13 May 1560).
31. Ibid., 67 (29 September 1565).
32. Ibid., 70 (12 January 1565/66).
33. Ibid., 175 (16 February 1582/83).
34. Ibid., 18 (26 March 1561).
35. Ibid., 69 (5 January 1565/66).
36. Ibid., 62 (25 November, 1564).
37. Ibid., 206 (6 April 1587).
38. Ibid., 64 (17 February 1564/65).
39. Ibid., 62 (14 October 1564).
40. Ibid., 103 (23 February 1571/72).
41. Ibid., 171 (28 July 1582).
42. Ibid., 10 (27 November 1559). The said child, Christian, was very successful at begging and that may have been a factor in the punishment of the mother. This 22d. collected in less than a week was a lot of money when one considers that Christ's routinely pensioned people at the rates of 6d. or 8d. per week.
43. Ibid., 110 (11 April 1573).
44. Ibid., 164 (27 May 1581).
45. Ibid., 71 (1 June 1565).
46. Ibid., 94 (3 June 1570).
47. Anne Somerset, *Elizabeth I* (New York: Alfred A. Knopf, 1991), 490.
48. Statutes of the Realm, 22 Henry VIII, A.D. 1531, chapter 12, in William Huse Dunham, Jr. and Stanley Pargellis, eds., *Complaint and Reform in England, 1436–1714* (New York: Oxford University Press, 1938), 423–29.
49. Allan, *Christ's Hospital Admissions,* 219 (25 April 1590).
50. Ibid., 5 (2 May 1558).
51. Ibid., 212 (5 September 1588).
52. Ibid., 14 (15 July 1560).
53. Ibid., 52 (30 October 1563). According to a footnote, he took a B.A. in 1581 and an M.A. in 1584; he became the vicar of Burford, Oxford, in 1600.
54. Ibid., 81 (29 November 1567).
55. Ibid., 61 (7 October 1564).
56. G.L., MS 12806/1, 4 September 1559.
57. Allan, *Christ's Hospital Admissions,* 2 (31 July 1557).
58. Ibid., 119 (13 February 1573/74).
59. Ibid., 17 (19 March 1560/61) and G.L., MS 12806/1.
60. Allan, *Christ's Hospital Admissions,* 100 (14 July 1571).
61. Ibid., 35 (10 April 1563).
62. Ibid., 32 (10 April 1563).
63. Ibid., 50 (7 August 1563).

64. Steve Rappaport, *Worlds Within Worlds: Structures of Life in Sixteenth-Century London* (Cambridge: Cambridge University Press, 1989), 298.

65. Salters' Company, Cl/I, fol. 37.

66. G.L., MS 12806/2, 31 March 1571.

67. Archer, *The Pursuit of Stability*, 157.

68. Firth, *Memoranda, References*, 83–84.

69. G.L., MS 12806/3, 19 February 1593/94.

70. Rappaport, *Worlds Within Worlds*, 295–96.

71. Ibid., 315–22

72. G.L., MS 12806/2, 16 March 1562/63.

73. Other professions include: founder, clothman, wine porter, instrument maker, brush maker, tapestry maker, dyer, hattbond maker, glover, innholder, packthread maker, shoemaker, painter, cutler, stationer, brown baker, brewer, scrivner, doctor of phisicke, bridle maker, skinner, chandler, leather seller, gentleman, labourer, tailor, point maker, fisherman, waterman, sailor, cordwainer, musician, mercer, vintner, tallow chandler, rope maker, blacksmith, haberdasher, anchorsmith, button maker, weaver, draper, girdler, joiner, ironmonger, goldsmith, silk weaver, salter, ministral, clothworker, cooper, and locksmith.

74. Allan, *Christ's Hospital Admissions*, 35 (10 April 1563).

75. G.L., MS 12806/2, 15 September 1571.

76. Allan, *Christ's Hospital Admissions*, 66 (18 August 1565).

77. Ibid., 36 (10 April 1563).

78. Ibid., 41 (10 April 1563).

79. Ibid., 34 (10 April 1563).

80. Ibid., 44 (10 April, 1563). *Wench* was not a derisive term but a commonly used Tudor expression for girl, much along the same vein as *lass* or *gal*.

81. Ibid., 208 (13 November 1587).

82. Firth, *Memoranda, References*, 83. Twenty-nine of Christ's children during 1552–98 were "preferred to university"; seventeen attended Cambridge, eleven attended Oxford, and one student's scholastic record has not been traced to either institution. George A.T. Allan, clerk of Christ's Hospital, edited the Children's Register in 1937 and traced these students through the universities and beyond. The cost of the higher education for some of these scholars was borne by outside agencies or individuals. Richard Dautrie was sent to Queens' College, Cambridge, by the Grocer's company, where he received a B.A. in 1575; he later moved to Peterhouse College (St. Peter's), Cambridge, receiving an M.A. from there in 1578. Thomas Colfe attended Broadates Hall, Oxford, due to the generosity of the Salter's company; he took a B.A. in 1581 and an M.A. in 1584. Walter Richardson's university costs were paid by the Fishmonger's company; he attended Christ's College, Cambridge. Edward Harrison was "Preferred to the University of Oxford by the Drapers," and took a B.A. in 1579. Anthony Dod was an alumnus of St. John's College, Oxford, through the auspices of the Goldsmith's company; he received a B.A. in 1578 and an M.A. in 1583. Roger Smith received a B.A. in 1581 and an M.A. in 1585 from Gonville and Caius College, Cambridge; his studies were supported by the Haberdasher's company. Gabriel Bowman and John Brigges received aid from the Clothworker's company; both attended Magdalen Hall, Oxford; Bowman took a B.A. in 1583 and an M.A. in 1587. Robert Chambers was a graduate of

St. Mary Hall, Oxford; he received a B.A. in 1586 and an M.A. in 1590, having been sponsored by the Vintner's company. Samuel Seedon was sent to university by the Ironmonger's company, but George Allan couldn't trace him through either Cambridge's or Oxford's records. In addition to guild support, university scholars could find assistance through the charity of individuals. Robert Cragge was sent to Christ's College, Oxford, by the earl of Leicester. A gift to the hospital from Mr. Dicksone enabled Daniel Hearne to earn a B.D. in 1614 from Peterhouse, Cambridge. The grammar master of Christ's Hospital, Mr. Waddington, sent Thomas Merrist to Gonville and Caius College, Cambridge. Merrist completed his B.A. in 1592 and a master's degree four years later. Additionally, William Harris took a B.A. in 1576 and an M.A. in 1579 from St. John's College, Cambridge. Thomas Austen completed a B.A. in 1585 at Magdalen College, Oxford. John Woodcocke took two degrees from St. Mary Hall, Oxford: a B.A. in 1582 and an M.A. in 1585. Richard Lane attended All Souls, Oxford and received a B.A. in 1590. Thomas Salisburie and William Clarke attended Peterhouse, Cambridge, the former taking a B.D. in 1621 and the latter taking a B.A. in 1617 and an M.A. in 1621. Although most of these students completed their studies and took a bachelor's degree, and many received masters' degrees, not all Christ's Hospital scholars took degrees at Cambridge or Oxford. John Uxleie, John Knightleie, George Cacie, William Lewis, and Richarde Marson either didn't take degrees or didn't stay long enough to enter into university records.

83. G.L., MS 12819/2, 29 September 1588–29 September 1589.
84. Ibid.
85. Allan, *Christ's Hospital Admissions,* 19 (23 June 1561).
86. Ibid., 34 (10 April 1563).
87. Ibid., 67 (30 August 1565).
88. Ibid., 64 (3 February 1564/65).
89. Ibid., 63 (30 December 1564).
90. G.L., MS 12806/2, 9 February 1571/72.
91. Allan, *Christ's Hospital Admissions,* 152 (23 May 1579).
92. Firth, *Memoranda, References,* 83.

Appendix A

1. G.L., MS 12819/2, 29 September 1596–29 September 1597.
2. Although common in Italy by the end of the fifteenth century, arabic numerals did not become common in England until the seventeenth century. See Frank J. Swetz, *Capitalism and Arithmetic: The New Math of the Fifteenth Century, including the Full Text of the Treviso Arithmetic of 1478,* trans. David Eugene Smith (La Salle, Ill.: Open Court, 1987), 290.
3. G.L., MS 12819/1, 23 June 1554.
4. WOULD YOU LIKE ME TO BE VERBOSE TODAY? (Y/N)
   ? y
   ACATES

   ACATES/MILK
   ACC.ADJUSTMENT

```
ACCOUNTBOOKS
ALDERMAN
ALE
ALLOWANCE
ALLOWANCE/RENT
ALMKEEPER/BETHLE
ALSM
ENTER DATE (0–31), OR 32 TO GO HOME, OR -1 TO GET LISTS OF
    CURRENT ITEM TYPES AND UNIT TYPES.
? 29
ENTER MONTH (0–12)
? 9
ENTER YEAR
? 80
ENTER ITEM DESCRIPTION (UP TO 16 CHARACTERS)
? writingpaper, etc.
HEY, THIS IS SOMETHING NEW! IS WRITINGPAPER, ETC
    CORRECT?
(Y/N/L-L WILL GIVE YOU A LIST OF ALL CURRENT ITEMS)
? y
PLEASE ENTER OLD ENGLISH PRICE NOW:
? vipviiis
+ 8. SHILLINGS =  .40 POUNDS
+ 6. POUNDS =  6.00 POUNDS
TOTAL PRICE =  6.40 POUNDS
HOW MANY?
? xviii
THATS   18 UNITS
ENTER UNITS (UP TO 16 CHARACTERS)
? ream/diversething
HEY, THIS IS SOMETHING NEW! IS REAM/DIVERSETHING
    CORRECT?
(Y/N/L-L WILL GIVE YOU A LIST OF ALL CURRENT UNITS)
? y
IS THIS A CREDIT (C), A DEBIT (D), OR A MISTAKE (M)?
? d
29 9 80 WRITINGPAPER, ETC 6.4000 18 REAM/DIVERSETHING D
ENTER DATE (0–31), OR 32 TO GO HOME, OR -1 TO GET LISTS OF
    CURRENT ITEM TYPES AND UNIT TYPES.
```

The prompts and program continues until issuing the "32" command at the end of an entry.

5. My computer figures do not gel with their figures. My totals for income and expenditures were tabulated through the addition of each separate entry. This is because I have tallied the figures for each calendar year and not for the hospital's fiscal year. Since Christ's Hospital had a floating fiscal year, it would be difficult to reprogram to accommodate their calendar.

6. Acates; acates/milk; acc.adjustment; accountingbooks; adjoininghouse; alderman; ale allowance; allowance/rent; almkeeper/bethle; alsm; annuity; applepies; apprentice; apron; areragis; armor; ashes; ashes/soap; assignes; assuranceoffice; attorney; baie/whitecotton; baiecloth; baiehall; baies; bailey; barber; barn&orchard, etc; barrelbutter; basket; bast; bay'swhite; bayliff; baysalt; beadle; bedding; beef; beef/mutton; beer; beer/bread; beer/carriage; bell; benevolence; bethlem; bill; billet; billet/carriage; billet/st.t; blackcap; blackcotton; blackfreise; blacklace; blacksmith; blackthread; blackwellhall; blanket; blk/chamberlain; blk/storehouse; blkhall/clerk; blkhall/collecto; blkhall/gallerie; blkhall/keeper; blkhall/library; blkhall/parson; blkhall/room; blkhall/surveyor; bluecloth; bluecloth/dressi; bluekersey; board; board/carriage; boardwages; boathire; bobbin; book; book/children; book/writingpape; books; bottles; boughes; bowes/broom; bowl/russes/stol; boxcomb; boxmoney; brasspan/cauldr; bread; bread/st.t; brick; brick/carriage; brick/gravel/sa; brick/sand; bricklayer; bridewell; broadbluecloth; broadquarterboard; broadwhitecloth; broom/roddes; broom/thread; broom/thread/ned; broomes; browncanvas; brush; buckle; building; burdeuxfeathers; burial; burialmoney; bushcoal; butter; butter/carriage; butter/cheese; buttery; caddas; calveskin/ cambridgestudent; candle/wick/ candles; candlestick; canvas; canvas/greencloth/ canvas/holland; canvas/lockeram; cappes; carmen; carpenter; carriage; carriageintocoun; carrotroot; carrots/pepper; casualreceipts; ch.warden/bread; chaffingdish; chamber; chamberlain; chamberoflondon; chandlor; changeofguard; charcoal; charges; cheese; cheese/carriage; chiefclerk; childbirth; childre; children/carriage; christ'shospital; churchwarden; churchyardcross; claretwine; clasps/hooks; cleaning; clerk; clerk-overseer; cloister; cloth; cloth/dressing; cloth/misc; cloth/dressing; clothing; clothworkers; clothworking; coal; coal/billet; coal/carriage; coal/smallcoal; coalhouse; coalhousekeeper; coarsecloth; coarseinckle; coat; collection; colliar; commonseal; commonseal/savoy; compter; construction; copy; cord; corkedshoe; cotton; cottoncandles; counsell; countinghouse; courtorder; coverlet; cowlstanes; curing; cushion; debt; debtpayment; debtrelief; debtremited; defenceinlaw; departing; diet; dinner; discharge; dishes; dishes/plates; dishes/platters; dispute; divinitystudent; doctor; doctor/curing; dowlas; dowry; dressing; dressing/trimmin; dublet; dutchfish; dutchherring; dutchwhitecanvas; dying; dyingofyarn; earthenpans; egg; elmtimber; enrolling; essexbutter; essexcheese; exchequer; extraordinarydeb; extraordinary; featherbed; fees; fellwool; ffrecis; finaltenement; fine; finecloth/dressi/ finedowlas/ finegreencloth; fineinckle;fiveweeks; flander'stowe; flax; fleecewool; fleetditch; foreverannutiy; forfeitleather; forfeyture; fourlazars; fourtennements; frame; freise; frouchers; fuel; fuel&coal; fulling; fulling/cloth; fulling/wool; gallery; garden; gardener; gentleman'sheirs; gentsholland; gift; girdles; glasier; glasslantern; goldsmiths; governor; governor/carriag; gracecloth; gravel; gravel/sand; grayfreise; greatcartcoal; greatcoal; greatcord; greathouse; greatlather; greatmadfish/st.; greatmesuage; greatoatmeal; greatpot; green'salley; greencloth; greencuslens; greenwadmoll; greenwoodmallin; grinding; grocer; ground; guild; guildman'sheirs; gutterstone; haberdashware; handmill/carriage; harford; hassock; heue/carriage/ hemp; herbes; herring; herring/carriage; herring/fish; herring/spratt; herring/st.t; hides; hogesheades; hollandcloth; hollandhempl hollandlinen; hollandlinge; honey; hoopes.labor; hooping; hooping/carriage; hor; horsehire; hosen; hosen/mending/ hosen/shoes; house; house&backside; house&gallery; house&garden; house&land; house&tennement; house&yard; income; incomereceipt; ink; ink/vessle; inkhorn; innsofcourt; install; installation; installoldstone; iron; ironmonger; ironwork; jacques;

jacques/hassock; hames; joyner; juniper; juyste/carriage; juste/powles; keeper; keepers/ lazarhou; keeping/child; keeping/lazar; keepint/sickman; keepingcourt; keepregister; kersies; king'sattorney; knight; knithosen; labor; labor/boathire; labor/stuff; labourer; lace; lading; lampoil; land; land&mill; landd&tennement; land&watermill; landpurchase; largetennement; laste/shoes; lathe; lathe/carriage; lathe/juyste; lawsuit; lazar; lazarhouses; lazarkeeper; lead; lease; leather; leather/carriage; leather/dressing; leathergirdle; leatherpoints; legacie; legalfee; lime;lime/gravel/sand; linen;linen/greencloth; linenyarn; livery; livery/nurse&mat; loan; lock/key; lock/ring/hook; lockeram; longcartcoal; lord'sheirs; lordwentworth; lynseiewolsey; mackarel; mackarel/carriag; maintenance; making; manchesterfreise; manor; mansion; marshland; mason; matron; matron/diet; matron/livery; matron/nurses; matron;'sdietmaid; meat; medow; mending; merchantadventur; mertement; milk; misc/acates; misc/buildingitm; misc/clothing; misc/ food; misc/householdit; money; money/borrowed; moneychangin; moneyleftover; moneyredelivered; morgan; morgan/diet; moskovatallow; mutton; n.cloth/dressing; n.gray/dressing/ n.kersy/dressing; nail; narrowbaie; necessaries; needleaccompt; needles; newbuilding; newcollection; newcountinghouse; newlandcod; newlandfish/carr; newstone; newtennement; nightcappes; normandycanvas; northerncloth; northerngray; northernpaling; northernrusset; northstraight; notary; nurse; nurses'livery; nursing; oaktimber; oatmeal; obligacon; offeringmoney; officer/c.h.; officer/c.h.&stt; officer/savoy; officer/st.t.; officers/c.h.; officers/st.t.h.; oil; oil/vessel; oilforlamp; oldcollection; oldlock&oldiron; oldrags; onelazar; onemonth; oneshovel; orchard&backside; ordinary collecti; overpayment; overseer; oxfordstudent; packthread; pail; painting/ painter; paper; paper/carriage; parch/quill/ink; parchment; quill; parish; parishcollector; parishpoor; paver; paving; payment; peason; peason/carriage; peastodds; pencion; pencions; penner/ inkhorn; pepper; perfume; petticoat; pewter; piece; pins; pins/needles; pipe; pipe/ carriage; pitchp pitch/tow; plain/greycloth; plainwhite; plankboard; plankboard/carri; plasterer; plasterer/brickl; platters; playse; playse/carriage; playse/fish; plumber; plummber/men; points; poor; poorpayment; poors'pension; poorwomen's gowns; portal; porter; portion; postfine; pot; powles; preparedocument; prerpgativecourt; prestaccount; printing; printinghouse; property; provisions; purchase; quarterboard; quarterboard/car; queen; queen'sbaylif; quirkset; quitrent; raisins; recompense; recorder; redherring; redlace; redlead; redspratt; redwax; relief; remembrance; rent; rent/parish; rentdue; rents; reparacion; reward; reward/alms; reward/curing; reward/matroon; reward/sickchild; reward/transfer; reward/wardens; roancanvas; roddes; rooftile; rope; rope/ pulley; ropes/pullies; rosen; rosetile; roughflax; roughtile; rubbish/carriage; rug; rushes; russetpetticoat; sack; salt; salt/carriage; saltbutter; sand; sandust; savoy; savoysurrender; saw; sawyer; scaffold; scholar; schoolhire; schoolhire/twowk; schoolhouse; seacoal; seacoal/ carriage;sewingthread;sexton/x'schurch;shoemaker; shoes; shoes/mendpetico; shop; shortflax; shorthemp. shovel; shrink/wet; sickchildren; sickward; sickwardrepair; silver/ sealc.h.; sirthomasramsey; skaffold/carriag; skinner'sshreds; smallbell; smallcoal; smalltennement; smalltong; smallyard; smith; smock; soap; soap.ashes.water; soap/water; soleleather; solicitor; soltewyche; sometimeannuity; sotheriebutter; soultege; sowther; spggot; spinningwheels; spittlesermon; sponge; spoons; spratt; st.barts; st.barts/ st.t.; st.thomashospita; stable; stable/roomes; stableroom; staff; stafftorch; stands/covers/ stanes; stationer; stationer; staywrit; stoolhemp; stopcock; storehouse; straw; straw/ carriage; strawhats; stuard; suffolk/dressing; suffolkbluecloth; suffolkbutter; suffolkcheese; surgeon; surplus; surreybutter; surreyland; sweetbutter; tallow; tallow/

carriage; tavern; taylor; teaching; tennement; tennement&garden; tennement&land; tennement&yard; thorncoal; thread; thread/ashes/soa; threehouse; threelazars; threetennements; threewarehouses; tile; tiler; tiler/plasterer; tilter; timber; timber/bell; timber/carriage; tinker; towe; towe/flax; townditch; trayes; treasc.h./st t.; treasurer/brides; treasurer/ch.h.; treasurer/st.bar; treasuar/st.t; treendishes; trenchers; tub/hooping/ twister/ cloister; twogardens; twohouses; twohouses&garden; twolaborers; twolazars; tworents; twosawyers; twotennements; twowarehouses; twoworkmen; tyler; tynne; uetthemp; unpaidobligation; unpaidrent; unreceiveddebt; usher; velum; viewday; vinegar; visiting; wage/diet; wages/ wages/fees; wainscot; ward/citizen; wardmoteenquest; warehouse; washhouse; washing; washingbetles; watchett; watchingcandle; water; water/ ladle/ water/physick; waterbearer; wateringpot; watermill&land; weaver; weaving/ weaving/hemp; weaving/linen; weaving/napkin; weaving/wool; weavin/yarn; week'sdiet; welchbaies; welchcotton; welchfreise; welchrug; well; estminster; wet/set/ whaleoil; wharfsage/carria; wheat; whipcord; white/wheatbread; whitebaie/cotton; whitebaies; whitebread;whitecanvas; whitecloth;whitecotton;whitegloucesters; whitegrasier; whitehartford; whiteherford; whiterowedplain; whiterug; whitesalt; whitesa;t/baysal; whitesalt/carria; whitethread; whitewelchcotton; whitewelshbaie; whiteynckle; whyting; whyting/carriage; wickcandle; widow; will; wiltshirewhite; windingsheet; windmill; wohall/baiehall; wohall/clerk; wohall/collector; wohall/keeper; wohall/parson; women; wood; wood/carriage; wood/coal; wool; woolencard; woolenyarn; woolenyarn/hosen; wooloil; workhouse; workman; workmen; worstedhall; writing; writingpaper; writing–paper, etc; writingschool; yard; yarn; yearlyrent; yeast; yeast/herbes; yncklecomb.

This program only accepts sixteen characters in a name and therefore some of these names seem odd because they have been abbreviated.

7. Food & drink; bookkeeping; clothing; apparel; cloth; income; fuel; St. Thomas; household item; bedding; blackwellhall; miscpayment; school; metal; legalfees; children; building item; labor; lighting; medical; other hospitals; staff; savoy & lazars; worsted hall; misc; grounds & buildings; pensions; nursing; necessaries; and rent.

8. Lotus 1-2-3. Lotus Access System V.lA (©), Lotus Development Corporation, 1983.

Bibliography

Manuscript Sources

GUILDHALL LIBRARY, LONDON

Christ's Hospital

12806/1	Court Minutes, 1556–63
12806/2	Court Minutes, 1562–92
12806/3	Court Minutes, 1592–1632
12812/1	Book of Legacies, 1592–1820,
12819/1	Treasurers' Accounts, 1552–58
12819/2	Treasurers' Accounts, 1561–1608
12818/1	Admission Register, 1554–99
12805	Register of Property, 1594
3339 (Box A)	"The Proseding at the funeral of Skynner esquier who died Lo. Maiore of London & was buryed as a barron."

Ward Records

4069/I	Cornhill Ward, Wardmote Inquest Book, 1571–1651

CORPORATION OF LONDON RECORD OFFICE

Rep. 13–28	Repertories of the Court of Aldermen, 1553–1609
Jour. 17–25	Journal of the Court of Common Council, 1555–1600

LIVERY COMPANIES

Salters' Company

C1/I	Ordinances, 1560–98

Books

Allan, George A. T. *Christ's Hospital Admissions*. Vol. 1, *1554–1599*. London: Harrison and Sons, 1937.

Archer, Ian W. *The Pursuit of Stability: Social Relations in Elizabethan London.* New York: Cambridge University Press, 1991.

Arthington, Henry. *Provision for the Poore.* London: Thomas Creede, printer, 1597.

Beaven, A. B. *The Aldermen of the City of London.* 2 vols. London: E. Fisher and Co., 1908–13.

Beier, A. L. *The Masterless Men: The Vagrancy Problem in England, 1560–1640.* New York: Methuen, 1985.

Beier, A. L., and Finlay, Roger. *London 1500–1700: The Making of the Metropolis.* London: Longman, 1986.

Blunden, Edmund, et al. *The Christ's Hospital Book.* London: Hamish Hamilton, 1953.

Boulton, J. P. *Neighbourhood and Society: A London Suburb in the Seventeenth Century.* New York: Cambridge University Press, 1987.

Bowden, Peter J. *The Wool Trade in Tudor and Stuart England.* Revised edition. London: Frank Cass, 1971. Originally published in 1962 by St. Martin's Press.

Braudel, Fernand. *Capitalism and Material Life, 1400–1800.* New York: Harper & Row, 1967.

Brigden, Susan. *London and the Reformation.* New York: Oxford University Press, 1989.

Carlton, Charles. *The Court of Orphans.* London: Leicester University Press, 1974.

Chambers, J. D. *Population, Economy and Society in Pre-Industrial England.* London: Oxford University Press, 1972.

Clark, Peter, and Paul Slack. *Crisis and Order in English Towns 1500–1700.* Toronto: University of Toronto Press, 1972.

———. *English Towns in Transition 1500–1700.* Oxford: Oxford University Press, 1976.

Clarkson, Leslie. *Death, Disease and Famine in Pre-Industrial England.* New York: St. Martin's Press, 1975.

Cressy, David. *Education in Tudor and Stuart England.* London: Edward Arnold, 1975.

Cunnington, Phyllis, and Lucas, Catherine. *Charity Costumes of Children, Scholar; Almsfolk, Pensioners.* New York: Barnes & Noble, 1978.

Davies, E. J. "The Transformation of London." In *Tudor Studies, Presented to A.F. Pollard,* edited by R.W. Seton-Watson. London: Longman, 1924.

de Mause, Lloyd, ed. *The History of Childhood.* London: Souvenir Press, 1976.

Dickens, A. G. *The English Reformation.* New York: Schocken Book, 1974.

Dickens, Charles. *Oliver Twist.* New York: Bantam Books, 1982.

Drummond, Jack C., and Wilbraham, Anne. *The Englishman's Food: A History of Five Centuries of English Diet.* London: Jonathan Cape, 1939.

Dunham, William Huse, Jr., and Parcellis, Stanley, eds. *Complaint and Reform in England, 1436–1714.* New York: Oxford University Press, 1938.

———. *Statutes of the Realm.* N.p., n.d.

Farjeon, Eleanor, and Farjeon, Herbert. *Kings and Queens.* Illustrated by Robin Jacques. London: J. M. Dent, 1983.

Finlay, Roger. *Population and Metropolis: The Demography of London, 1580–1800.* New York: Cambridge University Press, 1981.

Firth, J. F., ed. *Memoranda, References, and Documents Relating to the Royal Hospitals of the City of London*. London: Benjamin Pardon, 1803.

Flinn, M. W. *The European Demographic System, 1500–1820*. Baltimore: Johns Hopkins University Press, 1981.

Foster, Frank Freeman. *The Politics of Stability: A Portrait of the Ruler in Elizabethan London*. London: Royal Historical Society, 1977.

Fyfe, William Hamilton. "The Old Bluecoat School." In *The Barnwell Addresses*, vol. 2. Edited by John Louis Haney. Philadelphia: Mary Gaston Barnwell Foundation, 1937.

Gavitt, Philip. *Charity and Children in Renaissance Florence: The Ospedale degli Innocenti, 1410–1536*. Ann Arbor: The University of Michigan Press, 1990.

Goody, Jack. *The Development of the Family and Marriage in Europe*. New York: Cambridge University Press, 1983.

Grigg, David. *Population Growth and Agrarian Change: An Historical Perspective*. New York: Cambridge University Press, 1980.

Howes, John. *Contemporaneous Account, in Dialogue Form of the Foundation and Early History of Christ's Hospital and of Bridewell and St. Thomas' Hospitals*. Printed from the original manuscript of 1582 & 1587. London, 1889.

Hatcher, John, *Plague Population and the English Economy, 1348–1530*. London: Macmillan, 1977.

Jordan, W. K. *The Charities of London 1480–1660: The Aspirations and the Achievements of the Urban Society*. London: Allen & Unwin. New York: Russell Sage Foundation, 1960.

———. *Edward VI: The Threshold of Power, the Dominance of the Duke of Northumberland*. Cambridge: Harvard University Press, 1970.

Kahl, William F. *The Development of London Livery Companies*. Cambridge: Harvard University Press, 1960.

Kent, William, ed. *An Encyclopaedia of London*. London: J. M. Dent, 1970.

Kinney, Arthur F. *Titled Elizabethans: A Directory of Elizabethan State and Church Officers and Knights, with Peers of England, Scotland, and Ireland, 1558–1603*. Hamden, Conn.: Shoe String Press, 1973.

Kollock, Margaret R. *The Lord Mayor and Aldermen of London during the Tudor Period*. Philadelphia: John C. Winston,1906.

Macfarlane, Alan. *Marriage and Love in England: Modes of Reproduction, 1300–1840*. New York: Basil Blackwell, 1986.

McInnes, E. M. *St. Thomas Hospital*. London: George Allen & Unwin, 1963.

MacKenzie, W. Mackay, ed. *The Poems of William Dunbar*. London: Faber & Faber, 1971.

Nicholls, Sir George. *A History of the English Poor Law*,. New York: Augustus M. Kelley, 1967.

Nichols, John Gough, ed. *Chronicle of the Grey Friars of London*. London: Camden Society, 1852.

———. *Diary of Henry Machin, 1550–1563*. Camden Society Publication no. 42. London: Camden Society, 1848.

———. *Literary Remains of King Edward the Sixth.* Vol. 1. New York: Burt Franklin, 1964.

O'Donoghue, Edward Geoffrey. *Bridewell Hospital, Palace, Prison, Schools from the Death of Elizabeth to Modern Times.* London: John Lane, 1959.

Onions, C. T., ed. *Oxford Universal English Dictionary.* New York: Doubleday, Doran, 1937.

Outhwaite, R. B. *Inflation in Tudor and Early Stuart England.* London: Macmillan, 1969.

Palliser, D. M. *The Age of Elizabeth: England Under the Tudors, 1547–1603.* New York: Longman, 1983.

Pearce, E. H. *Annals of Christ's Hospital.* London: Methuen, 1901.

Pollard, A. F., ed. *Tudor Tracts 1532–1588.* New York: Cooper Square, 1964.

Pendrill, Charles. *Old Parish Life in London.* London: Oxford University Press, 1937.

Pollock, Linda A. *Forgotten Children: Parent-Child Relations from 1500–1900.* New York: Cambridge University Press, 1983.

———. *A Lasting Relationship: Parents and Children over Three Centuries.* Hanover, N.H.: University Press of New England, 1987.

Pound, John, *Poverty and Vagrancy in Tudor England.* London: Longman, 1982.

Priestley, Harold. *London: The Years of Change.* London: Frederick Muller, 1966.

Rasmussen, Steen Eler. *London: The Unique City.* Revised edition. Cambridge, Mass.: Mint Press, 1982.

Ramsay, G. D. *The City of London in International Politics at the Accession of Elizabeth Tudor.* Manchester: Manchester University Press, 1975.

Ramsey, Peter H., ed. *The Price Revolution in Sixteenth-Century England.* London: Methuen, 1971.

Rappaport, Steve. *Worlds Within Worlds: Structures of Life in Sixteenth-Century London.* New York: Cambridge University Press, 1989.

Simon, Joan. *Education and Society in Tudor England.* Cambridge: Cambridge University Press, 1966.

Skipp, Victor. *Crisis and Development: An Ecological Case Study of the Forest of Arden, 1570–1674.* Cambridge: Cambridge University Press, 1978.

Slack, Paul. "Mortality Crises and Epidemic Disease in England, 1485–1610." In *Health, Medicine and Mortality in the Sixteenth Century*, edited by Charles Webster. Cambridge: Cambridge University Press, 1979.

———. *Poverty and Policy in Tudor and Stuart England.* New York: Longman, 1988.

Stephen, Sir Leslie, and Lee, Sir Sidney, eds. *Dictionary of National Biography.* London: Oxford University Press, 1949–50.

Somerset, Anne. *Elizabeth I.* New York: Alfred A. Knopf, 1991.

Stone, Lawrence. *The Crisis of the Aristocracy, 1558–1641.* Abridged edition. New York: Oxford University Press, 1967.

Stone, Lawrence. *The Family, Sex and Marriage in England, 1500–1800.* London: Weidenfeld & Nicolson, 1977.

Stow, John. *A Survey of London.* Vol. 2. Edited by Charles Lethbridge Kingsford from the 1603 edition. 1908, rpt: Oxford: Oxford University Press, 1971.

Swetz, Frank J. *Capitalism and Arithmetic: The New Math of the Fifteenth Century, including the Full Text of the Treviso Arithmetic of 1478.* Translated by David Eugene Smith. La Salle, Ill.: Open Court, 1987.

Tawney, R. H. and Power, E. *Tudor Economic Documents.* Vol. 2. London: Longman, Green, 1951.

Thirsk, Joan, ed. *Agricultural History of England and Wales.* Vol. 4. Cambridge: Cambridge University Press, 1967.

Trollope, William. *A History of the Royal Foundation of Christ's Hospital.* London: William Pickering, 1834.

Twain, Mark. *The Prince and the Pauper.* New York: New American Library, 1964.

Unwin, George. *The Guilds and Companies of London.* New York: Barnes & Noble, 1966.

Weinreb, Ben, and Hibbert, Christopher, eds. *The London Encyclopaedia.* Bethesda, Md.: Adler & Adler, 1986.

Wheatley, H. B., ed. *Stow's Survey of London.* New York: Dutton, 1977.

Wheatley, Henry R. *London Past and Present.* Vol. 1. London: Singing Tree Press, 1968. Originally published in London by John Murraty in 1891.

Whitteridge, Gweneth, and Stokes, Veronica. *A Brief History of the Hospital of Saint Bartholomew's.* London: Governors of the Hospital of Saint Bartholomew, 1961.

Woodward, G. W. O. *The Dissolution of the Monasteries.* London: Blanford, 1966.

Wrigley, E. A., and Schofield, R. S. *The Population History of England, 1541–1871: A Reconstruction.* Cambridge: Harvard University Press, 1981.

Journal Articles

Beier, A. L. "Vagrants and the Social Order in Elizathan England." *Past and Present* 64 (1974).

Blanchard, I. S. W. "Population Change, Enclosure and the Early Tudor Economy." *Economic History Review* (1970).

Brown, E. H. Phelps, and Hopkins, Sheila V. "Seven Centuries of the Prices of Consumables, compared with Builders' Wage Rates." *Economica*, n.s. 23, no. 92 (1956).

Cornwall, J. "English Population in the Early Sixteenth Century." *Economic History Review*, 1970.

Cunningham, Carole. "Christ's Hospital: Infant and Child Mortality in the Sixteenth Century." *Local Population Studies* 18 (1977).

Harrison, C. J. "Grain Price Analysis and Harvest Qualities, 1465–1634." *Agricultural History Review* 19 (1971).

Hoskins, W. G. "Harvest Fluctuations and the English Economic History, 1480–1619." *Agricultural History Review* 12 (1968).

Kunze, Neil L. "The Origins of Modern Social Legislation: The Henrician Poor Law of 1536." *Albion* 3 (Spring 1971).

Te Brake, William H. "Air Pollution and Fuel Crises in Pre-industrial London, 1250–1650." *Technology & Culture* 16 (1975).

Index